Refugee Doctors

Support, development and integration in the NHS

Edited by

Neil Jackson

Dean of Postgraduate General Practice Education
London Deanery
Honorary Professor of Medical Education
Barts and the London

and

Yvonne Carter

Professor of General Practice and Primary Care and Vice-Dean
Warwick Medical School, University of Warwick

Foreword by

Dame Lesley Southgate

Radcliffe Publishing
Oxford • San Francisco

Radcliffe Publishing Ltd
18 Marcham Road
Abingdon
Oxon OX14 1AA
United Kingdom

www.radcliffe-oxford.com
Electronic catalogue and worldwide online ordering.

_____

British Library Cataloguing in Publication Data

A catalogue record for this book is available from the British Library.

ISBN 1 85775 857 9

Typeset by Aarontype Ltd, Easton, Bristol
Printed and bound by TJ International Ltd, Padstow, Cornwall

Contents

Foreword

Migration of doctors to seek additional opportunities for training and clinical practice is increasing and is part of globalisation. It is to be welcomed, although movement from parts of the world where there are not enough doctors to developed countries with very high standards of healthcare is, rightly, a matter for concern.

But this book is about doctors who have been forced to leave by circumstances beyond their control. Becoming a refugee – seeking asylum in another country, leaving hopes and dreams behind – is a profound trauma. The demonisation of asylum seekers, their shadowy images caught by infrared cameras as they try to cross borders, sometimes with children running beside them, should make us all reflect. In May 2004 there were 951 doctors on the BMA/ Refugee Council database, of whom 53 were working in the NHS, with a further 123 ready to apply for jobs. Some of these doctors might have been the same people caught on those cameras.

This book gives a very full account of many aspects of a complex situation. It details the history of refugee doctors and the range of problems they face, but it also shows the contribution that they can make and the personal courage and resilience it takes to survive the transition. Other chapters outline practical steps, from improving English to preparation for the examination they must pass and preparing for a job interview in a competitive market. The authors have all been involved in the process, either as refugees themselves, or as part of the widening group of professionals who are providing support and encouragement for these doctors.

I have chaired the Refugee Health Professionals Steering Group since its inception. We will have allocated about £2 000 000 of government funding to projects to facilitate refugee doctors' entry into the workforce. The money has contributed to doctors entering the workforce or being job-ready and is money well spent. It would have cost a great deal more to train a similar group of doctors from scratch and, in addition, there are people now working in the NHS who have come to share its values, and who are thankful for the opportunities they have been given to make a contribution. This book chronicles the progress we have made in our shared work to integrate these doctors. But it also demonstrates the need to continue, and to spread the approach to the needs of other healthcare professionals who are refugees and who wish to take a full part in British healthcare.

Professor Dame Lesley Southgate
Professor of Medical Education and Primary Care
Royal Free and University College Hospitals Medical School
May 2004

Preface

In the United Kingdom many refugees and asylum seekers have trained and worked as doctors, nurses, midwives and other professionals allied to medicine in the countries they have departed from. In the process of modernising the NHS workforce, with staff shortages in many areas, the skills of qualified overseas professionals are a valuable resource to be harnessed to the benefit of patients and local communities. The Department of Health (DH) has also fully acknowledged the invaluable contribution to be made by overseas-qualified professionals and in 2001 set up the Refugee Health Professional Steering Group with the task of overseeing DH funding and initiatives to support refugee health professionals in their efforts to seek employment in the NHS.

In addition, the Steering Group was formed to manage, co-ordinate and promote the programme of support outlined as recommendations in the government report published in November 2000, entitled *The Report of the Working Group on Refugee Doctors and Dentists*.[1]

Refugee health professionals are a cost-effective source of staff for the NHS in terms of retraining or integration into the workforce, as compared with the cost of training UK nationals. However, despite this, many refugees face considerable problems and difficulties in their quest to continue or resume their careers as health professionals in the UK. The DH Refugee Health Professional Steering Group has highlighted these as follows:

- difficulties with asylum applications
- difficulty in adjusting to 'training mode' which might be required to acquire registration in the UK
- previous interruption of training
- lost or destroyed documentation
- difficulty in securing references
- inability to speak English, if at all
- no contact with family members or other support networks
- difficulty in accessing appropriate information
- trauma experienced in their personal lives which has resulted in seeking refuge in the UK.

The needs of patients and local communities are paramount in the new NHS and must be supported by an appropriate system of planning, educating and developing a multiprofessional/multidisciplinary workforce of healthcare professionals at national and local levels.

The principles and values behind modernising the NHS workforce were set out in the consultation document *A Health Service of All the Talents: developing the NHS workforce* published in April 2000.[2,3] These included:

- teamworking across professional and organisational boundaries
- flexible working to make the best use of the range of skills and knowledge staff have
- streamlined workforce planning and development, which stems from the needs of patients and not of professionals
- maximising the contribution of all staff to patient care and doing away with barriers which say only doctors or nurses can provide particular types of care
- modernising education and training to ensure that staff are equipped with the skills they need to work in a complex, changing NHS
- developing new, more flexible careers for all staff
- expanding the workforce to meet future demands.

Other NHS stakeholder organisations and healthcare professionals have also actively addressed the modernisation agenda for workforce and development in the NHS. The NHS Executive (London Regional Office), for example, published a document of good practice for workforce and development in July 2000[4] which highlighted the kind of NHS workforce needed in London, i.e. one that:

- is equipped to recognise and meet the needs of the communities it serves and to reflect the nature of these communities
- is fit for practice and purpose, now and in the future
- is able to work in teams within and across professional and organisational boundaries
- is capable of sustained learning and development
- has easy access to appropriate knowledge and the facility to put this into practice.

The *Human Resources in the NHS Plan* policy document[5] takes forward the human resource commitments set out in *The NHS Plan*[6] to ensure that the NHS becomes a model employer offering model careers to NHS staff. *Human Resources in the NHS Plan* highlights four main objectives:

- making the NHS a model employer
- ensuring the NHS provides a model career through offering a 'skills escalator' (designed to offer NHS staff at all levels a means of career development and progression)
- improving staff morale
- building people management skills.

This book has brought together authors from varying organisations and professional backgrounds, all of whom are dedicated to supporting the integration of refugee doctors into the NHS workforce. The editors are particularly pleased to acknowledge the personal accounts given by two refugee doctors who describe their experiences in overcoming the obstacles and challenges required to succeed in working as doctors in the NHS (*see* Chapter 3).

It is intended that the readership of this book should extend to all healthcare professionals in primary and secondary care; NHS organisations including strategic health authorities, primary and secondary care trusts and other relevant NHS organisations. Most importantly, as editors, we hope it will guide and assist refugee doctors in the UK. In addition, it should act as a useful reference source to patients and lay members of the public working within the NHS.

The editors would like to record their thanks to Professor Dame Lesley Southgate for writing the foreword to the book and to our co-authors for their excellent contributions.

Neil Jackson
Yvonne Carter
May 2004

References

1 Secretary of State for Health (2000) *Report of the Working Group on Refugee Doctors and Dentists*. Department of Health, London.

2 Secretary of State for Health (2000) *A Health Service of All the Talents: developing the NHS workforce*. Department of Health, London.

3 Jackson N (2003) Work based learning and the retention and development of the NHS workforce. *Work-based Learning in Primary Care* 1: 5–9.

4 NHS Executive (2000) *Workforce and Development: getting people on board*. NHS Executive, London.

5 Secretary of State for Health (2002) *Human Resources in the NHS Plan*. Department of Health, London.

6 Secretary of State for Health (2000) *The NHS Plan: a plan for investment, a plan for reform*. Department of Health, London.

About the authors

The editors

Neil Jackson
Dean of Postgraduate General Practice Education, London Deanery, and Honorary Professor of Medical Education, Barts and the London, Queen Mary's School of Medicine and Dentistry, University of London.

Yvonne Carter
Professor of General Practice and Primary Care and Vice Dean, Warwick Medical School, University of Warwick.

The contributors

Sue Arnold
Assistant Director, Access and Development, North West London Workforce Development Confederation.

Michael Bannon
Director of Postgraduate Medical and Dental Education, University of Oxford.

Edwin Borman
Chair, Refugee Doctors' Liaison Group, International Section, British Medical Association.

Angela Burnett
Principal in General Practice and at the Medical Foundation for the Care of Victims of Torture London.

Sheila Cheeroth
Principal in General Practice and Clinical Lecturer (East London Refugee Doctors Programme), Barts and the London, Queen Mary's School of Medicine and Dentistry, University of London.

Diana Cliff
Refugee Health and Social Care Co-ordinator, North East London Workforce Development Confederation.

John Eversley
Senior Research Fellow, Department of Health Management and Food Policy, Institute of Health Sciences, City University, London. Research Consultant for various Refugee Health Professional Programmes.

Tony Fitzgerald
Programme manager, ESOL Barnet College, London.

Dilzar Razak Kader
Refugee doctor.

Anwar Khan
Principal in General Practice and Associate Director of Postgraduate General Practice, London Deanery, University of London.

Patrick Kiernan
Principal in General Practice and Course Organiser, St Mary's Vocational Training Scheme, North West London.

Sam McCarter
Lecturer in Academic and Medical English, Southwark College, London. Freelance writer and editor in Medical English and IELTS.

Jeanette Naish
Principal in General Practice and Senior Lecturer in General Practice and Primary Care, Barts and the London, Queen Mary's School of Medicine and Dentistry, University of London.

Geoff Norris
Course Organiser, Refugee Doctors' Clinical Experience Scheme, London Deanery, University of London.

Yong-Lok Ong
Associate Dean of Postgraduate Medicine for Overseas and Refugee Doctors, London Deanery, University of London.

Elisabeth Paice
Dean/Director of Postgraduate Medicine and Dentistry, London Deanery, University of London.

Jo Scrivens
Clinical Lecturer (East London Refugee Doctors' Programme), Barts and the London, Queen Mary's School of Medicine and Dentistry, University of London.

Zharghoona Tanin
Refugee doctor.

Penny Trafford
Principal in General Practice and Associate Director of Postgraduate General Practice, London Deanery, University of London.

Andrea Winkelmann-Gleed
PhD Researcher, Refugee Migration and Employment School of Development Studies, University of East Anglia.

Salt and stairs: a history of refugee doctors in the UK and the story of Dr Hannah Hedwig Striesow

Andrea Winkelmann-Gleed and John Eversley

'Thou shalt prove how salt is the taste of another man's bread, and how hard a path it is to go up and down another man's stairs.' (*Dante's Inferno* quoted by Norman Bentwich, writing about 1930s refugee scholars)

This chapter sets the contemporary experience of refugee doctors into a wider historical context. It focuses on the émigrés from Nazism and fascism in the mid-20th century. However, there are older examples of forced migration into Britain. For example, when Muslims and Jews were expelled from Spain and Portugal in 1492, some came to England. These Jews were later expelled (by James I) and then invited back by Oliver Cromwell. At the end of the 19th century there was another migration of Jews to England from Eastern Europe and the attitudes of some of the descendants of these communities towards the arrivals of Jews in the 1930s were significant, both in favourable and hostile points of view. Another example is linked to the expulsion of the Huguenots from France at the end of the 17th century, which brought another group of doctors to Britain. Out of these, nine were admitted to the College of Physicians in the 1680s. These migrants included not just doctors; John Dolland came to England as a weaver but later became an optician, joining his son to found the firm that still bears their name.

While recognising that the story of the internationally qualified doctors is one of migration and social historical events, it is important to be mindful that it is also one of individual, personal events which may or may not fit into common patterns. Thus the story of Dr Hannah Hedwig Striesow illustrates many of the wider patterns but also serves as a reminder of the individual identity of each migrant. This chapter draws on the experiences of Dr Striesow who fled to England in 1936 after having qualified as a doctor in Germany. Following her arrival in Britain, she was not allowed to practise as a doctor here until 1950. Her coping mechanisms and the story of her professional integration are illustrated; amongst other places, she worked as a nurse at the London Jewish Hospital. Following the recognition of her medical qualifications she worked as a GP in the East End for 40 years and was one of the first women GPs in Newham. In addition, she worked as a police surgeon and was the doctor in attendance at the Iranian Embassy siege.[1]

This chapter primarily addresses the experience of refugees who are already qualified or are nearly qualified. The evidence of previous generations of refugees is that both barriers and prejudice and eventual success are often passed on to subsequent generations born here or to refugees who came as children. The role of refugee doctors in supporting future generations should not be overlooked. Drs Muriel and Sammy Sacks, from refugee families themselves, produced four sons of whom three became doctors (including the well-known psychiatrist Oliver), but also helped later refugees such as Hedwig Striesow. Hedwig was also helped, through her husband who had been a student at the London School of Economics, by Prof Harold Laski, himself the grandson of a refugee and whose father and brother were heavily involved in healthcare for the Jewish community.

As modern refugee doctors struggle up the long stairs to recognition as professionals in the UK, this contribution might remind them that they have been climbed before and that salt sustains and enriches life in many ways, as refugee doctors have in the past and will continue to do.

Why refugee health professionals came to the UK

This chapter focuses on the refugees from Central, Eastern and Southern Europe before and during the Second World War, but they were not the first.

Jews and Muslims were expelled from Spain and Portugal in 1492. Among the Jews who came from Portugal was Rodrigo Lopez who became the Queen's physician. He was accused of poisoning her and even though the evidence against him was sparse, James I expelled him in 1609. Oliver Cromwell subsequently invited him back. The Huguenots were French Protestants who were expelled from France in the late 16th century. In the 19th century many Jews fled Poland and Russia to escape pogroms.

Refugees from Nazism, fascism and Stalinism

In the 1930s refugees from Nazism, fascism and Stalinism from all over Europe came to the UK. As well as Germany and Austria, refugees came from Italy, Czechoslovakia, Portugal, Spain, Russia and later Poland. Professor Josep Trueta, a distinguished surgeon, came from Spain for example.

In 1934 non-Aryan physicians in Germany were barred from participating in the state health insurance scheme. In 1937 Jews were no longer able to take exams to qualify as doctors. In 1938 all Jewish medical licences were revoked although some Jewish doctors were allowed to treat other Jews. Several estimates suggest that over half of Jewish doctors in Germany left the country in the 1930s. Medical students also applied to transfer their studies to other countries.

Between 1933 and 1935, 1200 academics were dismissed from German universities, of whom just over a third were from faculties of medicine. Among others who also had to leave was Albert Einstein. As well as Jews, colleagues who stood up for the rights of Jews and other groups and others perceived as having anti-Nazi ideas or lifestyles were dismissed. Some people were vulnerable to persecution for several reasons: Charlotte Wolff, for example, was a socialist, a Jewish doctor who set up the first birth control clinic in Germany and who made little secret of her lesbian sexuality.

Hedwig Striesow's (née Kohn) reasons for leaving Germany were essentially the fear of political persecution based on her ethnic identity, as well as her political beliefs. Hedwig's independence and strength of character were apparent from an early age.

'I had made up my mind to be a doctor when I was six and there was a saying in our family, I wanted to be a doctor like Dr Grünebaum who made my grandfather better. My grandfather died when I was eight.

I grew up in a boy's school; I was one of seven girls. Maybe that made me forget [that I was a girl].

I lived for a year with relatives when my mother died and then I lived on my own from 17 onwards.

I was in a very left-wing youth group; it was a very small group. It was a Jewish youth group – "Kameraden".

I very much considered to specialise in gynaecology, but I didn't. I hadn't got a choice. I wrote to [the German equivalent of the GMC], asking if I could practise as a doctor and they replied that under the present circumstances they would not consider. It said clearly because I am Jewish. I was very, very lucky that they let me finish my practical year; you had to have 12 months hospital experience before you were recognised.

It was getting more and more difficult and some people didn't realise what was happening. Some people said after the 1933 elections, it will all change again, the whole thing will be turned over again. I remember someone who had a small store in Nürnberg and the Nazis made it very difficult for him. He said, OK I close my shop and stay indoors and I am quite happy indoors – they killed him.'

How they got to England: the journey

To understand how refugee doctors in the 1930s came to England, it is necessary to understand not just the formal mechanics and policies but the underlying interests. Overall, refugees were not a government priority but civil servants and ministers saw that if the issues were not properly managed, it could become a major problem. They were therefore interested in the impact on the economy, public spending and international relations (with Germany and the Empire particularly). In relation to health professionals, while the government did not wish to antagonise the professions, it also saw refugees as an opportunity to enhance healthcare (particularly dentistry) and research. The effect of middle-class pressure for domestic servants, and professional objections to competition, meant that it was easier to come to England as a domestic worker than as a doctor. This led at least one doctor to propose coming to work as a butler, a proposal rejected by an immigration official on the grounds that 'Butlering requires a lifelong experience'.

The 1930s refugees generally needed sponsorship from someone in Britain and money to pay the German government in order to come to Britain. There was also a limit (set by the Nazi government) on how much money refugees could take out of Germany and this was further reduced in July 1934. Families, friends and colleagues were often the source of such sponsorship, but the Jewish community and organisations concerned with justice or human rights also helped out.

Hedwig's story highlights the importance of a support network in England and her sister had already set up residence here. She tells her story thus:

'I never called myself a refugee. I came to visit my sister; my boyfriend came before me. I came with a huge trunk; my boyfriend had a brother who looked like the Hitler Junge Quecks.* My (later) brother-in-law looked like this. So he took me to the ship, an English ship going from Hamburg to Hays Wharf in London. And my later brother-in-law took my luggage on board in Hamburg and said 'I am bringing this for a passenger'. Nobody looked at this blond young man taking my bicycle and the huge trunk in. I had a suitcase that the Nazis looked at. He reappeared and said to me 'Look at your pillowcase'.

---

* A book that was written about a German boy, who did everything for Hitler, who was blond and blue eyed.

He had put 300 marks in there. You were allowed to take 10 marks out or 20, I can't remember, 17 shillings.'

After the war started, there were many refugees from Central Europe all over the world. Despite a severe shortage of doctors in the UK, the Ministry of Health was reluctant to recruit them. From 1940 onwards, American doctors were recruited but, for example, a group of 80 Polish doctors stranded in Romania and a group in Shanghai were refused.

Professional attitudes to refugee doctors and its impact

Professional attitudes towards refugee doctors have not been uniform either at a particular time or at different periods. For example the College of Physicians welcomed Huguenot physicians in the 1680s, but were more restrictive towards migrant doctors in the 1930s and 1940s (see below). In the 1930s the difference in attitudes towards internationally qualified doctors among various professional bodies was particularly significant. Within the BMA alone, there were a variety of attitudes. In 1934, the Chairman (Brackenbury) and Secretary (Anderson) of the BMA said there would be no opposition to the entry of doctors fleeing the Nazis as long as they did not go on from Britain to any of the Dominions (South Africa, Australia, New Zealand, Canada) where there was opposition from their members.

Within the Medical Practitioners Union (MPU), there was even more open and virulent opposition. The MPU was a much smaller, grass-roots organisation than the BMA and many MPU members felt that the BMA did not reflect their views and interests. These issues included state-sponsored medicine. They felt that financially the panel system was driving them into debt and forcing them to practise a kind of orthodox medicine that they did not wish to practise. For example vaccination and vivisection were central issues. A fascist group got into senior positions in the MPU with a Bethnal Green GP, Maurice Beddow Bayly, prominent among them. The MPU journal he edited blamed Jewish banks for the debts of GPs and said that the asylum-seeking doctors would be a further threat both in their numbers and how they would practise. The MPU views found expression in BMA conference motions so that the number of refugee doctors that the BMA agreed with the government was reduced and also the doctors were interned along with other enemy aliens though they were released shortly after. After the war, the MPU tried unsuccessfully to have the refugee doctors expelled.

The Royal Colleges of Physicians and Surgeons were also more hostile than the BMA to admitting refugee doctors. The President of the Physicians was Lord

Dawson. His attitude to refugee doctors from Germany is important because it demonstrates very clearly the interplay between politics, bureaucracy and medicine. Dawson's professional life was spent at the London Hospital. He was the author of a famous report in 1920 that anticipated the organisation of the National Health Service. Based on his experiences as a major general in France in the First World War, he advocated the formation of a health service based on the distinctions between primary, secondary and tertiary care. He was also physician to the King and friend of politicians, including Lloyd George, who was also his patient. In 1936, he, Lloyd George and a civil servant working closely with the Prime Minister of the time, Baldwin, spent two days with Hitler. According to his biographer, Dawson was very interested to see if the 'eugenic enterprises of national socialism could ... provide lessons for Britain in the drive for national fitness'. Although Dawson entertained refugees at his dinner table in Wimpole Street and helped many of them to start their life and work afresh, his basic stance was unhelpful. At a meeting with the Home Secretary in November 1933, he said of refugee doctors that: 'The number that could be usefully absorbed or teach us anything could be counted on the fingers of one hand'.

Even in 1938, professional leaders were still saying 'British medicine has nothing to gain from new blood and much to lose from foreign dilution'. In the light of this and also Nazi ideas about 'Aryan' and 'Jewish' blood, it is particularly fitting that refugee doctors such as Walter Weiner and Otto Leyton made significant contributions to establishing the Blood Transfusion Service (BTS), often considered to be a quintessentially British innovation.

Arrival: establishing themselves professionally and personally

Personal settlement

The refugees who arrived in 1933 or soon after generally settled in London in the middle-class suburbs, avoiding the East End Jewish communities with whom they did not closely identify, in many cases. Later on there was more dispersal as sponsors tried to find places for the refugees.

For most of the first 10 years Hedwig was in England, her accommodation was tied to her work as a nurse, which created many restrictions for her personal life, something not unusual in those days.

In 1939, Hedwig had to stop working at the London Jewish Hospital because aliens were not allowed to work in hospitals assigned for military casualties as the London Jewish then was. 'The new matron, she was very good, she said "Until you find somewhere to live, you can stay in the Nurses' Home as my guest, but don't enter the hospital itself"'.

When Hedwig moved to Lingfield Hospital in Surrey, she was also given exceptional help: 'The matron said that they had built a new house for her and that we could have the old matron's flat'.

For some adults (3000 in September 1939) their first home was a former army training camp ('the Kitchener') at Richborough in Kent run by the Council for German Jewry. Among them were 80 medical doctors. The BMA would only permit those with Italian qualifications to treat even fellow inmates.

Although a few enemy aliens were interned in 1939, larger numbers were not interned until May 1940. These included refugee doctors who were allowed to treat fellow internees, the first opportunity for many to practise since coming to England. At Onchan camp on the Isle of Man, there were 38 physicians among nearly 1500 inmates.

Altogether, 27 200 men and women were interned and 7350 were deported to Canada and Australia. Some particularly unlucky internees were put on the ship the *Arandora Star* to be deported to Canada, but the ship was torpedoed in July 1940, resulting in the drowning of 650 people. Among those on board was an Italian gynaecologist, R Vicchi-Borghese, who survived. The internment policy was reversed in July 1940 and some of the deportees returned to the UK. Other internees who joined the Pioneer Corps, where they were used as manual labourers, got early release.

Max Glatt, the psychiatrist whose work is discussed further below, endured several of these arrangements. Having qualified and practised in Germany, he was imprisoned there several times. He was interned in Dachau concentration camp but released and with difficulty made his way to England. Then between 1939 and 1940, he was in the Kitchener camp and from 1940 to 1942 he was interned on the Isle of Man. Finally in 1942, he was deported to Australia. Later in 1942 he came back and started working as a medical officer in Surrey.

Hedwig's story illustrates the internment policy further, as her husband was among the first to be interned.

'My husband, being non-Jewish, having a father as a captain in the German merchant navy – not a very good recommendation – was interned. He was sent to the *Arandora Star* where enemy aliens were interned to go to Canada ... As a married woman, if my husband wanted to go to war, I had to give permission. Well, I wasn't going to give permission. So I said, "I refuse to give permission to my husband to leave Britain". So he ended up on the Isle of Wight [interned] for about a year. Laski helped get him out of internment.'

Establishing themselves professionally

In 1935, the British universities said that they did not have any places for refugee medical students. The Home Office said that even if they got places, they would not be permitted to remain in the country. In all, 75 or fewer students, partially trained in the UK, were finally allowed to practise in 1940 on a temporary basis. More who had all their training in the UK were allowed to practise without limit. By July 1938 only 264 non-nationals had been admitted to the register.

Most of the doctors who had already qualified had to sit the Scottish triple or Conjoint examination – the final medical exam for students outside the universities. Dawson thought it alarming that this route was used and tried to get the Home and Scottish Offices to make the Conjoint Board raise the admission requirement. Some were able to sit the shorter exam for refugee doctors in London. Colleges for the refugees formed themselves – a Polish medical college in Edinburgh, a Czech one in Bristol.

By 1935, 125 of the doctors had already got recognised qualifications with 41 still completing courses. Most were in general practice as principals or assistants.

Hedwig did not even try to get recognition as a doctor when she first arrived as she felt that this would be futile. For 17 years she mostly worked as a nurse, first at the London Jewish Hospital and then at Lingfield in Surrey and then back at the London Jewish as a night sister. It is very clear that the experience of nursing gave her opportunities to improve her English, her knowledge of UK healthcare practice and, crucially, professional contacts, as well as an understanding of British society.

> 'I didn't contact the General Medical Council. I thought it was hopeless. I knew it on the grapevine. My sister probably knew some people who had tried it. Looking back, I should have smuggled more money out of Germany. I wasn't unhappy as a nurse, funnily enough; some people were terribly unhappy, I wasn't.'

The London Jewish Hospital knew she had trained as a doctor.

> 'Once I was established after the first few months, they said, well you know what to do, but I never took advantage of it with the other nurses there. I must have been there about four months, they said "Give Mrs X an enema" and I said, "Sister, I don't know how to give an enema". She looked at me and said, "I thought you are a fully trained doctor!" I said, "Yes I am, but that doesn't fall into a doctor's curriculum". That was a rather big joke, which went round the hospital. I had become a nurse, wiping people's bottoms. I wasn't the only doctor who came and there was one who came after me who had practised as a doctor for 12 years and was much older than me and he had to work as a probationary nurse.
>
> When I saw a nurse doing it incorrectly I would say, "Can I help you?" They said, "What's gone wrong?". They were glad that they got out of trouble; they would have had to go to the sister and explain.'

Hedwig moved to Lingfield Hospital in Surrey. Again, the move reflected the importance of professional and personal contacts.

In 1939 the government established a register of specialist skills (of British and foreign persons) and 1940 an International Labour Branch. Many doctors not already recognised were allowed on the Temporary Register for the Emergency Medical Service established in 1941. However, restrictions (formal and informal) were put on where they could practise. By 1944 over 3000 alien doctors were on the register. Jut over a third were in civilian employment. The vast majority were attached to British or allied armed forces.

The arrival of Hedwig's children meant that she had to change her working pattern.

'After I had my children I went back to work. I did some manual work and I did some translation then. I went to work after my second child. The London Jewish Hospital was in terrible trouble, short of night staff. I don't know what happened to the night sister, something happened. They absolutely needed relief for the nights, "Six nights on and 18 nights off, would you be interested?" I said, "What do I do with my baby?" "Bring it." So I brought him, he stayed in the Nurses' Home at night; I fed him when I arrived and I fed him before I left. My husband looked after the older one. In my spare time, I knitted for people.

I had learned to get on with uneducated people probably as a nurse. It probably made me a better doctor, because some things they will tell a nurse, they won't tell a doctor – could make a lot of difference. I could swear like them. I could say, "Bloody hell, I don't want to deal with that". I learned to communicate with patients from having been a nurse, probably much better than you would as a junior doctor.'

At the end of the war many of the doctors attached to armed forces were repatriated. Some of these doctors clearly saw themselves as being in temporary exile from occupied countries or serving their country from outside. However, the government plan during the war had been that many of the others would be repatriated too. However, the Home Secretary in the newly elected Labour government (James Chuter Ede) realised this was politically and practically impossible. His civil servant representative on the aliens committee noted not only that some refugees had been in England for over 10 years but also many would dread going back and would not be made welcome. Furthermore, the National Health Service was about to be created and there was an overall shortage of doctors. Nevertheless, when some employment restrictions were explicitly lifted on refugees in 1945, the restrictions on doctors and dentists remained. What they were not told was that there was no legal basis for these continuous restrictions. Eventually in 1948 the GMC's permanent register was opened to refugees and 1000 refugee doctors went on to it after that. However, those with previous well-established careers as specialists and consultants found it very hard to get posts of similar status. The major exception to this was the psychiatrists from Continental Europe who had a much more established system of education, training and specialist development in mental health than Britain.

As far as it is possible to estimate, it appears that just under half the 500 or so 1930s refugee doctors practising in 1945 were practising in London. Many had general practices that included a high proportion of refugees.

Hedwig's decision to resume her medical career was encouraged by one of the consultants at the London Jewish.

> 'One of the consultants at the London Jewish said it is ridiculous that you work here as a nurse if we could have you as a doctor. I needed four. I didn't have to do anything, just six months' probation. I had my exam results and I also wrote to the university [in Germany] to get them to confirm that I had passed the exam and I got some papers. I was lucky that I had brought out all my course papers. Registration took a long time. You had to fill in pages and pages. I think it asked "Why did you come here?". I probably said it was rather dangerous being member of a socialist students movement and being Jewish. They didn't test my clinical skills. I think the consultants were asked about my English and how I got on with patients. They asked that in the recommendation. They interviewed me.'

Hedwig was invited to apply to take over a general practice in Newham. The interview for the practice seemed more interested in her status as a woman doctor than as a refugee.

> 'I was at the London Jewish on my probationer year when the practice came up. The practice was after all written out for a woman. The Women's Voluntary Service asked for it to be a woman. They said it was a working-class area.
>
> When the practice came up they said, we might cut your probationer year. I was only eight months in or something. [The consultant at the London Jewish who was her guarantor] told me I wouldn't get it. I didn't have the right background.
>
> I had the interview in Piccadilly and when I applied I thought, I haven't got a chance, there will be so many people applying, but it won't do me any harm to get the experience of an interview. I had put on my best-tailored costume; I had my hair done (it was a great expense for me, but I wanted to look a professional person). They asked me why I wanted to work there. I think it was because 90% of German Jewish refugees lived in Hampstead and Golders Green. They asked how I would cope with a family and what attitude my husband would take. He was an enormous support, he was a partial invalid. He did a lot of my written stuff. I said he would support me in every way. They asked a lot of questions, what attitude I had to abortion, etc., was I interested

in obstetrics? They asked what would I do if I had male patients with specifically male problems; would I catheterise a male . . .?

I was completely by myself. I had to go to a police station here and ask which was actually East Ham, and the next corner is West Ham. And then came the next difficulty. I had to find a place to practise in within 30 days. Do you know what the housing situation was like in 1950? It was like asking, can I move into Buckingham Palace? There were no houses for sale, no houses to rent, there was enormous shortage, no rebuilding yet. I needed money to buy a house and the consultants of the LJH all pulled together with a loan giving a guarantee of £300 and £50 each.

I officially retired when I was 80, but then I was my own locum for quite a long time because we couldn't find a suitable successor. So I retired in 1988. I carried on seeing some private patients for a time.'

The 'objections' to refugee health professionals practising

Language, culture and communications

The view that refugee doctors would not be able to communicate properly had been expressed before the Second World War. MS Holzman of Palestinian and Australian background was refused admission to the London Hospital in 1927 for training because he was 'too curt'. He was helped by Redcliffe Salaman who advised him that:

'Much weight is placed in this country on good, not to say facile, manners . . . little things [are disliked], such as sitting down in a room before you are asked to; not getting up when the owner of the room or the responsible person comes in; answering questions curtly, and without an occasional "Yes, Sir" which is often most resented.'

After the war, British diplomats in the Near and Far East tried to interest government departments in the UK in bringing refugees to Britain. However, the departments resisted this on grounds of English language difficulties and international qualifications being hard to verify. This affected a number of doctors and nurses who sought refuge in Shanghai. Finally India agreed to accept some of them.

There could be language problems. The story is told of two famous refugee psychiatrists in the United States struggling with the pronunciation of a key concept for a lecture. Their eventual choice of penis 'envoy' rather than 'envy' caused much laughter. Hedwig recognised that there were communication problems.

'I had taken some English lessons before I came but my English must have been horrible. I wasn't the worst. A large number of patients spoke Yiddish, which I never spoke. I once went to Berlin and there was a Yiddish-speaking community but I had never heard or spoken Yiddish before. I managed to communicate with the patients somehow. It was quite funny sometimes. I was too well integrated already. I was the doctor with the funny accent. It was a deliberate decision of mine not to lose my accent. If someone doesn't want to have anything to do with me, keep out. I took some grammar lessons because I wanted my written work to be perfect.

The English nurses called the German Jewish nurses in the hospital rude and bad mannered. Generally the German Jewish nurses came from an upper-class background, so why were we rude? One day I got very annoyed and asked why are we rude and ignorant? You call us that and I didn't know why. Out it came, we didn't say "excuse me" when we went out of a room and closed the door. When we had a [bread] roll we didn't cut it, we broke it. They were odd things like this; they thought we were ignorant and they were educated because they cut their roll. It was silly things.

Standards

Lord Dawson, whose position was described earlier, justified it by saying that while he had 'the greatest respect for the German pioneers in medical science . . . he considered that the German methods of teaching and approach had fundamental defects'. Dawson said that under the German system, 'The patient is apt to be regarded as a piece of machinery, resulting too often in a callous disregard for the feelings and sufferings of the sick'.

Hedwig noticed similarities and differences between her training and that of UK-trained doctors. Despite social medicine being more advanced in Germany than in the UK, it had not been a compulsory subject for her, for example, and she learned its importance from experience.

'They didn't know how to mix syringes. I had learned it at university. You learned to cope, you learnt to improvise. I came from a very good background. The medical training essentially it wasn't different. It took me a long time to understand how difficult working conditions were for some people. I had a patient who spent years at the port and couldn't use either his left or right arm properly. I explained to them that he was quite OK to do hard work, but he couldn't do fine mechanics, but any heavy work was not beyond him. They came back and asked if he would be on probation for another post and I said that he would do his best to keep his job, he did. It would sometimes be possible to transfer from a cutting job to a sewing job, in a gown shop.'

Competition

The views of the MPU in the 1930s and 1940s have already been outlined but the view was much more widespread that students and professionals from refugee backgrounds were unfair competition for British doctors. The BMA feared that letting the doctors practise might 'take the bread away' from British doctors on war service and this view carried on within the NHS. While there was an overall shortage of doctors, the system of progression and promotion meant that refugee doctors with specialist backgrounds were competing for jobs with non-specialist UK-trained doctors whom appointment panels preferred.

Public and patient hostility

The belief that patients would find refugee doctors unacceptable was widespread in the 1920s and 1930s. The Chief Medical Officer, Arthur Newman, held this view.

In a prolonged argument about whether refugee status in the UK should be temporary or permanent, public opinion was regularly cited by both government and by Anglo-Jewish representatives as a reason for making it temporary. Herbert Morrison, the Home Secretary, repeatedly argued that allowing the refugees to gain citizenship would lead to outbursts of anti-semitism and public disorder.

Although these public views may have been present in the media and policies towards refugees, they did not always filter through to the grass-roots level and some refugees remained unaffected by such hostilities. Hedwig didn't experience them directly.

'I didn't have any negative reactions. They already saw that I had a strange name; those who didn't want me, didn't come near me, I hope. I don't remember any difficulties. One of my sons came home once and said that somebody at school was nasty, but I didn't send them to private school, they went to the local school. He learnt to defend himself, he was OK afterwards.

It was easier to integrate then than it is now. I mean, nobody expected me to go to the pub every night but when I came in, I was always made to feel welcome. I had quite a few pub keepers on my books. If you did a visit there, [the invitation] to "come in for a drink" was automatic. I got an awful lot of respect. We used to be invited to weddings, christenings, funerals and it didn't matter what religion they or you were. I tried to avoid it as much as possible but on the other hand I would probably go to the church when they got married and then disappear. I wanted to show that I was friendly but on the other hand you probably knew hardly anybody there and I had enough work.

I had a lot of Jewish patients, about a third of the population here were Jewish. I had a lot of Irish but I really can't remember the first coloured patients that I worked with. There were one or two Indians there. Very gradually that changed. The Indian men liked when their women had a woman doctor and I made it clear that I preferred to have families register, not single members of a family, so the men came as well.

I remember somebody from some organisation asking, "What did I think of the colour question?" and I replied, "I was persecuted by the Nazis. Can you imagine my position?". I happened to have a friend who was married to a Nigerian, a very impressive Nigerian, and they saw him going in and out of the house and it all made a difference.'

Fear that refugee health professionals were physically or mentally ill

One of the objections to (even training the children of) refugees and immigrants has been the claim that they are dirty, unhygienic or diseased. The Chairman of the London Hospital Governors claimed that one of the Jewish students had gonorrhoea and syphilis. It sparked a debate about whether to admit more students of refugee origin. Today, assertions about HIV or hepatitis among refugee health professionals are similarly stereotypical.

Personal attitudes, values, beliefs

In the 1920s students of Russian Jewish origin were sometimes discriminated against because of presumed Communist sympathies.

Jewish applicants for medical school after the Second World War were regularly asked if they were Orthodox Jewish on the assumption that if they were, they would be unwilling to attend patients on a Saturday.

Major Greenwood, from the London School of Hygiene, who was treasurer of the Academic Assistance Council helping refugee scholars, probably reflected the stereotypical view of many colleagues when he praised the research skills of the refugee doctors but opposed them practising because of an 'excessive sense of self-importance'.

Relationships between colleagues

Discrimination by colleagues was often explicit, sometimes 'justified' by alleged patient attitudes. In the 1920s and 1930s, the BMJ regularly carried adverts saying 'No Jews or Men of Colour' when advertising general practice vacancies and quotas and exclusions were widely apparent in hospitals. Jewish and refugee students at Barts on the eve of the Second World War had to endure anti-semitic graffiti and a fascist student magazine justifying persecution in a 'Poem to Hitler'.

Hedwig found colleagues supportive: 'One of my colleagues was very help-ful. He was a Scottish Jew and he was just a nice person and helped when I needed advice'.

Professional careers of refugee health professionals in the UK

Hedwig made a number of distinctive professional contributions as a police sur-geon, in setting up an out-of-hours rota in Newham and through her interest in maternity services.

> 'Somebody said to me, we haven't got any female police surgeons around here, go and apply for it. I did an exam in Germany in forensic medicine in 1933; it was one of the subjects you could choose. And do you know a polite way in England to say "no"? I got a letter from Scotland Yard saying, "Thank you very much, but we have no vacancy, if ever should one occur, we might get in contact". Very polite way of saying "no". But about six weeks later at evening surgery when I still had very few patients, the telephone rang: "Can I speak to a doctor? This is the Metropolitan Police, could the doctor possibly go to West Ham, there is a man at the station who thinks his wife is dying and he wants a doctor urgently".'

Having correctly identified an illegal abortion as the cause of death, Hedwig became a female examiner for sexual offences.

> 'I was the doctor in attendance at the siege of the Iranian Embassy. They asked, could I come and I came and I stayed until it was over because I was a police surgeon. When it was all over they cooked us a meal, I think it came from one of the Hyde Park hotels.'

Hedwig was also responsible for setting up an out-of-hours duty rota among GPs in Newham and a GP-led maternity unit.

Impact on patients and medicine in Britain

The contributions that refugee doctors have made to medicine in the UK reflect a number of different ways in which the fact of being a refugee or a migrant might have added value. Some already had established skills when they arrived or came from a tradition that was underdeveloped in the UK. Others were able and highly motivated. Because of the block on opportunities to go into popular specialties, some of them went into neglected clinical areas or research.

Some refugee doctors have taken a particular interest in health issues relevant to the communities they are from, often addressing prejudice and discrimination in the process. In the 1920s the Jewish Health Organisation undertook research demonstrating that eye problems among Jewish children were the result of genetic predisposition rather than caused by excessive Hebrew study. Hugh Gainsborough and Otto Leyton pioneered work on diabetes; both identified problems and solutions because of its prevalence in the Jewish community. Leyton began the manufacture of insulin when it was not readily available in the UK and introduced modern blood transfusion methods to the UK.

Others brought new skills and techniques. Josep Trueta's experience of treating victims of aerial bombing in Barcelona led him to develop closed plaster treatment for wounds and broken bones. Dr Guttman, a refugee neurologist, pioneered work with men with spinal injuries at Stoke Mandeville Hospital in Buckinghamshire, establishing it as an international centre of excellence.

The contributions of the refugee scientists to research have been phenomenal. Refugees who came to the UK in the 1930s included at least three Nobel Prize winners for medicine (Ernest Chain, Hans Krebs and Bernard Katz) as well as one for chemistry (for Max Perutz for his work on metabolism) that was of profound significance to medicine. Josef Rotblat received the Nobel Prize for his work on nuclear weapons but went on to become Professor of Medical Physics at Barts. By 1953 there were eight refugee medical researchers who were Fellows of the Royal Society (FRS).

Refugees, notably within mental health and neurology, established whole branches of medicine. Sigmund Freud (and his daughter Anna) helped establish psychoanalysis. Before they came, few people were practising psychoanalysis. One of the few was David Eder who came from a refugee family but also was a leading light in the Jewish Medical and Dental Emergency Association. Many refugees went into psychiatry. Max Glatt, who pioneered the rehabilitation of people with alcoholism, was working in a back ward of a mental institution and while chatting to some alcoholic patients, discovered they were bored with making elephants in the occupational therapy centre. He went on to found a unit for alcoholism and drug addiction at St Bernard's Hospital in Ealing and later worked at University College Hospital. He never retired and worked until shortly before his death at 90, in 2002. Joshua Bierer, an Austrian, pioneered work with therapeutic groups and therapeutic communities at the Runwell and Marlborough Day Hospitals. Erwin Stengel's studies at Sheffield added significantly to understanding suicide. Sidney Bloch, who came from Hamburg in 1936, was one of the founders of the Psychosomatic Research Society. Felix Post came from Germany in the early 1930s while still a medical student. He pioneered old age psychiatry in the UK but did so almost unwittingly.

'I thought Aubrey Lewis [the consultant] wanted me at the Maudsley ... because of my brilliant promise. Later on it became clear that he was thinking of having a department for old age psychiatry, for which he had earmarked me. He never told me this, which is maybe just as well.'

Michael Balint was Hungarian born, a trained doctor and psychoanalyst who fled in 1939 because of anti-Semitism. His approach to listening to patients, and GPs sharing experiences, has had a profound effect on general practice in the UK.

Robert Steiner started his medical studies in Germany, finished them in Dublin and went on to develop radiology, particularly magnetic resonance imaging (MRI) in London.

On the other hand, specialisms that could have been reinforced and invigorated were not because of restrictions. Public health, social medicine and occupational health were all very strong in Germany but a whole cohort of doctors was denied opportunities in the UK and went to the USA instead. Restrictive British policy had one positive effect on occupational health, however. Rudolf Laban, the dance choreographer, was unable to find enough work in his chosen field so he went to work for the Mars confectionery company and other manufacturers where he helped them improve the posture of their operatives, pioneering the introduction of ergonomics in industrial production.

Settlement in the UK: personal developments and identity

Name changes

The history of refugee doctor settlement is peppered with those who have (generally) anglicised their names though it is not the norm.*

Some did so to avoid hostility at times of conflict: Professor ASF Grunbaum (1869–1921) was a cancer specialist. He was professor of pathology and dean of the Medical School in Leeds and changed his name to Leyton in the First World War. Otto Fritz Grunbaum (1874–1938) also changed his name to Leyton in the same period. He was a physician and scientist at the London Hospital in the 1920s and 1930s. The Dean of Westminster Medical School, Adolphe Abrahams, advised at least one prospective student to change his name.

---

*One of the authors' own family name (Eversley) is a translation of his refugee father's German name (Eberstadt) with the added delight that it is also the anglicised name of a 17th-century Huguenot refugee doctor's family (Lefevre).

Some have done so to celebrate their acceptance as professionals in Britain: the writer on philosophy, Brian Magee, recalls Dr Perkoff in Hoxton changing the sign outside his surgery from Perkoff to Perkins on getting his British nationality.

Hedwig was called Hannah after her arrival in England. She resumed calling herself Hedwig early in the 21st century.

'I prefer to be called Hedwig, because Hannah was my Hebrew name. Hedwig was so difficult and when I got naturalised, I adopted Hannah. My birth certificate is "Hedwig".

I was a great supporter of the war, as you can imagine, having lost not only my job, my profession, [having] relatives killed. My most exhilarating moment was when we beat the Nazis. I am a Labour Party member. I joined it here in Newham as soon as I could afford the fees. I am socialist.

When I was working as a night sister, I attended a religious service perhaps twice a year when I was in London. In the 1930s and 1940s I occasionally accompanied my sister to a service in London. But I was not particularly interested. I didn't light candles on Friday night. I was inactive. During Passover I didn't give up bread. I wore sleeveless dresses. I had breakfast, bacon with my breakfast, I still have but I never broke the rules while in the hospital. Because if you commit yourself to work in a nunnery, you are not bringing boyfriends in. What I did outside of the hospital that was my affair, but while I was inside I respected the rules, but with common sense. I remember one occasion when I revolted against it; a patient had suddenly collapsed on Sabbath, I can't remember the details and I said, we must ring his relations. And they said, you can't use the telephone; I said, "That's an emergency, I will use the telephone".

I have never been one inclined to pray, it took me a long time to realise what prayers could do to people. I belong to a Jewish community now, the congregation I joined now, more for a decent cremation than anything else. Funnily enough, the rabbi there is the son of a co-student of mine.'

Attitude to subsequent refugees

Support for the refugees of the 1930s came significantly from earlier generations of doctors from a refugee background. The Jewish Medical and Dental Emergency Association was an offshoot of what had become the London Jewish Medical Society but had formerly been the London Jewish Hospital Society. By March 1934 it was estimated by the Association that there were 180–200 refugee doctors.

The Society for the Protection of Science and Learning (created in 1937 out of the former Academic Assistance Council) excluded Jews from its Council in order to emphasise that discrimination against academics was general but also to avoid anti-Semitism. Jewish support was given discreetly.

It has been argued that the health and careers of some refugee doctors suffered because of the support that they gave others. However, the health and careers of many refugee doctors suffered for many other reasons too.

Hedwig helped launch a campaign by the BMA to support modern refugee doctors and continues to observe the situation of refugees.

'I have little to do with refugees now, but before it was educated refugees who came to England, it's probably a broader [range] now. We expected very little help and I think expectations now are bigger and it's right, for more help to be given. I agree with it, but it makes it difficult. The immigrant people are keeping to themselves and you have to argue against that. I think the quicker one integrates into the population the better. There is more hostility than probably we got. We were looked at more as a curiosity.

Context

This handbook focuses on the immediate context for refugee doctors. There are two historical observations that may put the situation into a broader perspective.

The first is from Lord Goodman. Arnold Goodman was a lawyer and adviser to the British Prime Minister, Harold Wilson. He was seeking to explain why so many second-generation Jewish immigrants and refugees went into medicine. He said: 'Most Jews . . . have their bags packed, metaphorically speaking, and a medical degree is highly portable'.

However significant the obstacles to recognition for refugee doctors are now, it is worth remembering that medicine is not only a more portable skill than many others but it is becoming more portable as both illness and learning become more internationalised.

On the other hand, it is also salutary to remember what happened after World War I. During the war medical education had been opened up to women and people from poorer and immigrant backgrounds, because of the shortage of middle-class men. After the war, prestigious medical schools closed their doors to these newer entrants. Lord Knutsford of the London Hospital Medical School famously justified the exclusion of women because of the effect it had on the school's sporting achievements but he also said: 'In view of the drain caused by the war the hospital had been accepting for some time past students of various nationalities and creeds of a different type and of a different social standing to those formerly received and the experiment had not been successful'.

We must make sure that removing the barriers to recognition of refugee doctors is not seen as a temporary expedient at a time of labour shortage or an experiment that 'failed'.

Reference

1   The material on Hedwig Striesow is based on a series of interviews conducted by Andrea Winkelmann-Gleed and John Eversley during 2002 and 2003. A fully referenced version of this chapter is available from the authors.

Further reading

- Bentwich N (1953) *The Rescue and Achievement of Refugee Scholars: the story of displaced scholars and scientists 1933–52.* Martinus Nijhoff, The Hague.

- Cooper J (2002) *Pride Versus Prejudice: Jewish doctors and lawyers in England, 1890–1990.* Litman, Portland, Oregon.

- Honigsbaum F (1979) *The Division in British Medicine.* Kogan Page, London.

- London L (2000) *Whitehall and the Jews.* Cambridge University Press, Cambridge.

- Mosse WE (ed) (1991) *Second Chance: two centuries of German-speaking Jews in the United Kingdom.* JCB Mohr (Paul Siebeck), Tubingen.

- Shorter E (1997) *A Short History of Psychiatry.* Wiley, New York.

- Strauss H and Roeder W (eds) (1983) *International Biographical Dictionary of Central European Émigrés. Volume II, parts 1 and 2.* KG Saur, Munich.

- Watson F (1950) *Dawson of Penn.* Chatto and Windus, London.

- Wilkinson G (ed) (1993) *Talking about Psychiatry.* Gaskell, London.

- Wilson F (1959) *They Came as Strangers.* Hamish Hamilton, London.

CHAPTER I

Refugee doctors in the UK

Edwin Borman

Introduction

'Refugee doctors want to contribute to the society that has given them sanctuary, not depend on it.' That message is frequently heard from doctors seeking asylum in the United Kingdom who often have arrived with little more than the clinical knowledge they carry in their minds. For the medical profession they present a challenge: to assist with the integration of these colleagues. For the UK they represent a marvellous opportunity; at a time when the NHS needs more doctors, they bring their qualifications and expertise for free. It makes both humanitarian and economic sense to help refugee doctors re-establish their careers in this country.[1]

These messages have been supported by many individuals and organisations keen to help these doctors. There has also been some assistance from government, including the provision of financial resources for projects in this area. In England this money has been distributed by the Refugee Health Professionals Steering Group (RHPSG) established by the Department of Health (DH).

This follows work previously carried out as part of the DH's human resources responsibilities. A working group of the Overseas Doctors Sub-Group of the Advisory Group on Medical and Dental Education, Training and Staffing (AGMETS) published its report on refugee doctors and dentists in November 2000.[2] Its recommendations included:

- the establishment of a voluntary database of medically qualified refugees
- an information pack for medically qualified refugees
- support from postgraduate deaneries
- clinical attachments to be provided free of charge
- the General Medical Council (GMC) to waive the costs of the first two attempts at the tests required for registration

- the GMC to defer the costs of registration itself until refugee doctors have taken up employment.

Initial difficulties

The problems faced by individual refugee doctors can be overwhelming. To settle in a new country is never easy; to do so having had to flee one's own is even harder. Many doctors have escaped political or social persecution, some have been victims of torture. The psychological effects of these may profoundly affect any attempt at re-establishing their careers.

In the UK the Home Office is responsible for assessing asylum claims, a process that despite recent changes may be protracted. This and the nature of the process itself are major sources of anxiety for doctors. Should they be granted asylum through one of a number of potential categories, the applicant is then formally termed a refugee. Immigration policy has always been a contentious political issue and the UK government's policy of 'dispersal' has meant that community support – well established in the London area – cannot be relied upon elsewhere for individuals who may often be vulnerable. Efforts continue to be made to provide adequate assistance in the 'cluster' areas to which asylum seekers and refugees have been dispersed.

Maslow's hierarchy provides a clear indicator of the basic needs that must be met – food, clothing, housing – before higher needs such as education can be practicably embarked upon.[3] It is essential therefore to ensure that links are developed between those wanting to assist refugee doctors with their careers and bodies that are specialised in supporting essential needs.

Individuals and organisations that want to help refugee doctors also face major problems. Local or regional projects find it difficult to obtain resources for an issue that many do not regard as a high priority. Until recently they may also have been limited by the lack of co-ordination and expertise required to establish supportive programmes.

A template to identify and address needs

Those working in this area have developed a template to identify the essential components of a comprehensive and integrated programme that is matched to the path that refugee doctors will take towards employment. This is based on eight stages:

- identification on joining a programme
- the provision of information
- a first phase of orientation

- preparation for required assessments
- the examinations themselves
- a second phase of orientation
- registration in the UK as a medical practitioner
- competition for a job.

Efforts to achieve greater integration of projects that support refugee doctors have been facilitated by the Refugee Doctor Liaison Group (RDLG) hosted by the British Medical Association (BMA).

Identification

While many may have given up hope of practising as doctors in their adoptive home, word of mouth and information provided by the Refugee Council ensure that refugee doctors find their way to supportive programmes. On doing so they are invited to provide their details for a voluntary national database maintained by the BMA; Figures 1.1 and 1.2 provide recent information from this.

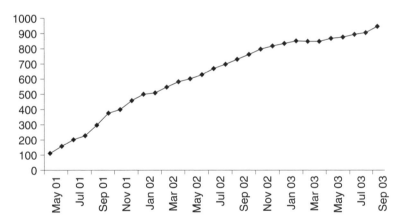

Figure 1.1 Month-on-month increase of doctors on the Refugee Doctors' Database

Northern and Yorkshire	87	West Midlands	75	Eastern	16	Wales	18
North West	103	Trent	49	Scotland	39	London	517
South East	29	South West	10	Northern Ireland	0		

Figure 1.2 Location of refugee doctors in the UK, September 2003

Similar databases have been established by local and regional projects. These ensure that doctors are linked to a wide network of supportive organisations and that those providing support can attempt to match resources to needs. Comparison of databases reveals that up to 40% of doctors actively working to re-establish their medical careers have yet to join the national database; these figures may therefore underestimate their true number.

Information

It is essential that doctors are provided with the information necessary to guide them through what for UK-trained doctors is a complex system, but for refugees can be intimidating. It is necessary for them to contact many organisations – covering matters ranging from language to medical training and registration – each of which provides information relevant to its own responsibilities. There had been little attempt to combine the information provided until recently when, as part of the work co-ordinated by the RDLG, the Jewish Council for Racial Equality (JCORE) published the first *Refugee Doctors' Handbook*. This is now made available to all doctors who join the national database.

To provide information on a more regular basis, the BMA publishes a quarterly Refugee Doctors Newsletter, again mailed to all doctors on the national database. This includes a list of useful websites and up-to-date information on national and regional initiatives. The BMA also makes available to refugee doctors a package of benefits that includes free copies of the *British Medical Journal* and access to the BMA library.

Orientation

Preparing to take the initial steps in an unfamiliar cultural and professional environment can be daunting. At the same time many doctors have unrealistic expectations of the timescale and extent of what they will be able to achieve. To provide guidance at this crucial stage, many local and regional projects provide support in the form of mentoring, needs assessment and/or careers guidance.

Each of these is a highly intensive process based on one-to-one communication; ideally it also involves regular opportunities for review. To make this possible some projects have developed networks of established or retired doctors familiar with the UK system who have volunteered their time and efforts. The Refugee Education and Training Service (RETAS) of Education Action International has been funded to assist with the training of mentors. An alternative and innovative means of addressing these issues is the 'buddy system' being developed in Oxford that links refugee doctors and final-year medical students.

Preparation

To be eligible for registration, refugee doctors are required by the GMC to demonstrate their competence in linguistic abilities and their medical knowledge and skills. This almost always involves preparing for and achieving the required scores on the International English Language Testing System (IELTS) examination and passing the two Professional and Linguistic Assessment Board (PLAB) examinations.

Many refugee doctor projects provide support for doctors studying for some or all of these examinations. Typically this would be in the form of language classes for doctors preparing for IELTS, the latter part conducted in advanced, hence more cost-intensive classes. Work carried out at Southwark College indicates that on average it takes two years for someone who has come to the UK with little knowledge of English to pass IELTS at the high language standard required of doctors.[4]

There are many commercial courses assisting doctors who want to prepare for the PLAB examinations; because of their cost these are out of the reach of any refugee doctor. Specific courses have therefore been established by projects wanting to assist refugee doctors in this area. These include North Central London College, which provides PLAB 1 and 2 teaching by lectures and a distance learning programme;[5] the Refugee Doctors Programme at St Bartholomew's and the London hospitals that, in addition to assisting doctors to pass the PLAB examinations, equips them with the skills required to succeed in their medical careers;[6] and the West Midlands PLAB 2 course, which has a remarkably high pass rate.[7] It is clear that many advantages can be achieved when projects are structured or combined to support doctors 'seamlessly' through their preparation for IELTS, PLAB 1 and PLAB 2.

Examination

The IELTS examination is administered by the British Council and tests doctors in four components: reading, writing, speaking and listening. The GMC requires a minimum average score in the IELTS of seven from doctors who plan to sit the PLAB examinations, with a minimum score of six on the listening, reading and writing and seven in the speaking components (seven is classified as 'good user'). The £73 cost of the examination is paid by some supportive projects for refugee doctors who have shown in language classes that they have reached the required standard and have a reasonable chance of passing.

The PLAB examination is controlled by a board accountable to the GMC. As a generalisation, PLAB 1 focuses mainly on medical knowledge while the PLAB 2 examination assesses medical skills and communication. Both require of the refugee doctor a significant element of adaptation to the relevant knowledge base and the cultural context of medical practice in the UK. The GMC itself has waived the £145 cost of the first two attempts at part 1 of the PLAB examination for refugee doctors who provide the required evidence, but doctors sitting the PLAB 2 examination still have to find the £430 cost for this. Again, some projects will provide this funding subject to their own satisfactory assessment of the refugee doctor's likelihood of passing the examination.

Orientation

Having passed the required examinations, doctors may begin looking for employment. The GMC requires this to be in a supervised post, hence almost always in the NHS. For many refugee doctors the manner in which medicine is practised in the UK is considerably different from that with which they are familiar. A second phase of orientation frequently is helpful, including clinical attachment(s) with supervising consultants, learning about the actual workings of a clinical team.

Clinical attachments tend to be in an observership capacity, with few or no 'hands-on' responsibilities. Guidelines on these have been written by Cheeroth and Berlin and are available on the BMA website.[8] These emphasise their educational content and the responsibilities of all parties, and have been supported by the GMC and the DoH. The GMC also accepts references from clinical attachments of more than six weeks' duration.

A number of regional postgraduate deaneries provide assistance with finding clinical attachments, mainly through keeping a database of consultants and general practitioners willing to provide these. Deaneries also provide 'Recruitment and Induction' seminars, a further form of orientation that usually includes an introduction to the NHS, advice on the preparation of a curriculum vitae and interview skills.

Registration

The GMC requires satisfactory completion of the IELTS and PLAB examinations and confirmation of a job offer before granting registration to a doctor. This will be limited registration and satisfactory reports on their progress will need to be provided to the GMC by doctors when they apply for full registration. Some doctors prefer to apply for Pre-registration House Officer (PRHO) rather than Senior House Officer (SHO) posts, believing this to be a more satisfactory means of entering the UK training grade structure.

As always, costs can be prohibitive. The current registration fee in 2004 is £290 with a further £100 for scrutiny prior to this. To assist refugee doctors, who are likely still to be surviving on benefit payments, 'interest-free' loans are provided by some projects in which the money required for initial registration is repaid when the doctor has begun working.

Competition

While locum employment may be attractive, doctors are encouraged to seek substantive posts that are fully recognised by the deanery. The advantages of this are that these posts will always be accepted by the GMC, are likely to provide better training and should be compliant with hours-of-work regulations.

While there remains a general shortage of doctors at all levels in the UK, this is not always the case in certain specialties and in some parts of the country. Refugee doctors are therefore encouraged to apply for posts that may not be their first preferences, as obtaining their first job and references is more important to their future career than waiting for the 'right' job. The London Deanery recognises this in its small scheme of funded posts specifically tailored for refugee doctors on the basis of providing much-needed preparation through work experience.

Projects do not subscribe to positive discrimination, preferring to ensure through thorough preparation that 'their' doctors will be 'the best person on the day for the job'. Figure 1.3 shows the self-reported figures from the national database of doctors who, in less than three years, have made major progress and are providing an example for colleagues to follow.

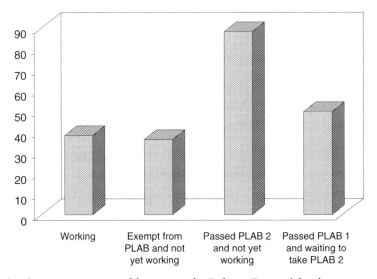

Figure 1.3   Career progression of doctors on the Refugee Doctors' database

Lessons for the future

A number of key points can be derived from the experience of those active in supporting refugee doctors.

There are considerable advantages to be gained from integration. This can be 'vertical integration' in which a project or a group provides support covering all elements of the template described above: from first identification of the refugee doctor to their successful appointment to a medical post. Birmingham, Glasgow and London provide well-developed examples of this. The pan-professional approach taken by projects, 'horizontal integration', permits the sharing of resources and costs; it also introduces individual healthcare professionals to teamworking of a nature that will be fundamental to their future NHS practice.

The successes that can be achieved are considerable. Individual doctors have succeeded in ways that have surpassed their expectations and those of their supporters. While each of these certainly can be seen in humanitarian terms, there also are economic advantages. The NHS currently is suffering the effects of a well-documented shortage of doctors at all career levels; the integration of refugee doctors provides a potential resource of highly motivated and skilled professionals. Early analyses support a 're-qualification cost' of around £6000 for a refugee doctor, a fraction of the £200 000 required for a doctor to graduate from a UK medical school.

The need for resources is perpetual. While new projects still struggle to find initial funding, more established ones have difficulties achieving continued funding, despite having overcome start-up costs and being able to demonstrate successful outcomes. The DH in England over three years has provided £1 500 000 distributed through the RHPSG;[9] smaller sums have been provided in Scotland and Wales to support projects in these nations. A general trend away from these centralised forms of funding suggests that in future projects will have to compete for 'mainstream' funding from workforce development confederations, primary care trusts and strategic health authorities.

Innovative working is a remarkable characteristic of refugee doctor projects. The combination of motivated individuals and organisations working in unorthodox teams, having to cope with limited financial resources while drawing on considerable educational knowledge and communication skills, has produced results that potentially have far wider applicability. A further characteristic is the willingness with which such expertise is shared.

Conclusion

The limitations of this short chapter mean that only some of the many projects and organisations that are active across the UK can be mentioned. Where initially there were few, now there are many providing creative ideas on how the needs of refugee doctors can be met. They are achieving results that have been described as a 'win-win-win': doctors are able to progress with their careers, patients and the NHS benefit from their expertise and society is provided with a positive example of what the refugee community can bring.

The integration of refugee doctors in the UK provides a successful model that already is being applied to other health professionals and, with small adaptations, could be applied outside the healthcare sector. When so many countries appear increasingly reluctant to provide sanctuary, this also presents an opportunity to challenge ill-informed ideas.

References

1   Adams K and Borman E (2000) Helping refugee doctors. *BMJ.* **320**: 887–8.

2   Department of Health (2000) *Report of the Working Group on Refugee Doctors and Dentists.* Advisory Group on Medical and Dental Education, Training and Staffing, Overseas Doctors Sub-Group. Available at www.doh.gov.uk/pdfs/refugee.pdf.

3   Maslow A (1954) *Motivation and Personality.* Harper, New York.

4   McCarter S (2003) Personal communication.

5   www.plabisgood4u.com

6   www.birminghamplabcourse.com

7   www.smd.qmul.ac.uk/gp/refugeedoctors

8   www.bma.org.uk/ap.nsf/Content/ClinicalAttachmentGuidelinesIntro

9   Department of Health (2003) *Integrating Refugee Health Professionals into the NHS.* Refugee Health Professionals Steering Group. Available at www.doh.gov.uk/medicaltraining intheuk/pdfs/sgreport.pdf.

CHAPTER 2

Getting refugee doctors back to work: the challenges, obstacles and solutions

Yong-Lok Ong, Michael Bannon and Elisabeth Paice

The challenges and obstacles

The precise number of medically qualified individuals who hold refugee status is unknown. Estimates based upon the practical experience of those who have tried to help them back to work within the NHS vary between 200 and 2000. A self-registering database is now maintained by the Refugee Council jointly with the British Medical Association and this exercise should yield useful information in terms of demographic details, previous levels of skills and expertise and preferred career aspirations in the UK. The phenomenon of refugee doctors is not new, however. Previous eras of conflict have resulted in large numbers of professionals in all disciplines seeking refuge in the UK and other countries.[1] Experience to date would strongly endorse the very positive contributions that refugees have made in their new countries.[2,3] The plight of refugee doctors has attracted considerable attention more recently, both from the media[4] and from the medical press.

There is added value in integrating refugee colleagues into the NHS. They bring with them considerable and unique skills, many of which are valuable in a multicultural society such as ours. They have already graduated from a medical school and many will have completed postgraduate specialist training with transferable skills. While acknowledging the need for further support in order to work in the UK, many refugee doctors are already partially trained. It would seem good sense to take advantage of their previous experience while there is a chronic shortage of medical skills in the NHS.

The reality is somewhat different and depressing. Numerous accounts exist of the struggles encountered by refugee colleagues in their attempts to gain employment as doctors. Until recently, relatively few managed to achieve this aim. The accounts given reveal an apparent uphill struggle at every step. Refugee doctors would appear to be a valuable resource in a country chronically short of doctors. It is frustrating to everyone, not least themselves, that their return to practice should be so fraught with problems.

Comparison with other overseas doctors

In comparison with refugees, other overseas doctors seem to have it easy. The situations are different in many ways, however, and the special challenges in employing refugee doctors need to be thoughtfully recognised and addressed, not ignored.

The challenges can be categorised as lack of the following:

- documentation
- professional support
- established career pathways
- knowledge of the system
- fit between skills and NHS needs
- ability to communicate in English
- experience of working in a multicultural society
- financial resources
- psychological support
- mutual trust and understanding.

Most overseas doctors coming to train in the UK have planned for the event for some time. They will have spoken to colleagues who have had training in the UK, looked up websites and researched the training system. There may be links between their institution and one in the UK and they may have been selected for UK training by their institution as part of a well-trodden pathway. They will certainly have ensured that their English language skills are up to working in the NHS. They may be supported financially from home or go straight into well-paid training posts on arrival in the UK.

In contrast, refugee doctors are unlikely to have planned for working in the NHS. When refugees leave their country, it is often under conditions of extreme secrecy, haste or stress. They may not have brought the documentary evidence to prove their medical qualification or any postgraduate degrees they may have acquired. They are unlikely to be able to produce references. Their institution may not be familiar to potential employers. Some may have excellent English but many have little or none. Overseas doctors usually have, in our experience, adequate levels of medical English and may have used English-language texts in their undergraduate education. Their refugee colleagues may speak little or no English and are likely to have studied medicine in their own language.

Most overseas doctors come to the UK at an appropriate point in their training to benefit from the further training on offer in the NHS. Refugee doctors have little choice about when they come. As a result they are often older than the average trainee and grow older still as they struggle over hurdles such as PLAB and IELTS. The consciousness that time is passing and that younger doctors are progressing in their careers while they are being left behind is painful, especially if – as is often the case – they have held senior positions in their home country. Frustration may become resentment, bitterness or even despair.[5]

Table 2.1: Differences between refugee doctors and other overseas doctors

Overseas	Refugee
Prepared to come to UK	May not have prepared
Know what to expect	May not know what to expect
Have necessary documents	May not have documents
Have recent references	May not have references
Planned departure	Traumatic departure
Coming for training	Coming for refuge
Usually recent experience abroad	May not have worked for some years
Usually 29–39 age group	Wide age range
Likely to have some funds	Likely to be very hard up

Employing refugee doctors and risk management

Health systems are very different as is the epidemiology of diseases in different countries. Much of the knowledge and many of the clinical skills acquired in the home country may be only marginally relevant in the UK. To cite a few examples, a refugee doctor from Africa had worked mainly in African villages and gained detailed knowledge of dealing with malnutrition and parasitic infestations but only had basic information gleaned from textbooks of other medical conditions. Of two Middle Eastern doctors, one was highly proficient in dealing with trauma cases as a result of war injuries and the other was skilled in desert medicine, treating scorpion and snake bites. Both were less sure of dealing with the common medical conditions seen in the UK. Even professional values and attitudes differ between countries, especially with regard to patient choice, multiprofessional working and attitudes to women. During interactive sessions in induction sessions, male doctors have expressed the view that their word should not be challenged by patients or other members of the team as they are in a position of authority. Interestingly, it is not uncommon for female doctors during these sessions to report that their male colleagues and fellow countrymen persist in perceiving their medical roles as being less important because they are women.

All of these potential problems are only too well known to NHS employers. They make employing a refugee doctor seem a risky proposition in comparison with a UK graduate or an overseas doctor who can demonstrate fluency in English and familiarity with the UK system.

There will also be worries about clinical risk, especially in terms of prescribing practices, clinical procedures and communicating with colleagues, all of which may have been very different in the home countries.

There will also be worries about 'fitting in'. How will a doctor who may have come from a tight-knit unicultural environment fit into a multiethnic, multicultural and multiprofessional team dealing with the extraordinarily diverse population that makes up a city like London? Additionally, some refugee doctors may have been leaders of their professions in the home country. Their high profile may have put them particularly at risk of persecution. For such a high achiever, it may be extremely difficult to adjust to working at a lower level, perhaps having to take orders from a younger and less experienced doctor or being criticised or corrected by nursing and other colleagues in the multiprofessional team.

Box 2.1: Case study

These difficulties are clearly illustrated by the vignette of a refugee doctor who had achieved the position of specialist psychiatrist in his motherland. At age 47 after being out of medicine for five years, he was offered a supernumerary SHO placement. Having been assessed in this role and found to be satisfactory, he was then appointed as a substantive SHO on a psychiatric rotation in open competition. This appointment was made in the trust where he had been a supernumerary. As a substantive SHO several difficulties occurred. His supervising consultant and college tutor felt that problems were caused by his reluctance to consider the views of the multidisciplinary team. His defence was that they were not medically trained and many were younger and not even English. He dropped out of the rotation with plans to join a GP training scheme where he hoped he would have more autonomy. He is presently unemployed.

Given their experiences, refugee doctors may continue to suffer fears for themselves and their families even in the apparently safe haven presented by the UK.

Feelings of paranoia and rejection are understandable. It is easy for these to be directed at the employers who are seemingly so unfairly reluctant to give them a chance. Embitterment is destructive[7] and trust takes time and familiarity to develop.

What is needed is a system that allows refugee doctors a chance to demonstrate their capabilities and their readiness to learn and adapt without undue delay after they have passed the necessary tests of clinical and linguistic skills. Such a system should be low risk, moving from theory to practice, from hands-off to hands-on, at a pace dictated by the individual and his or her needs and above all by the needs of the patient. Some projects that have set out to do just this have been completed and the rest of this chapter will be devoted to their description.

Clinical attachments

Clinical attachments are well established as the way for overseas and refugee doctors to gain experience of the NHS and to obtain a reference.[8] An unpaid clinical observership offers the opportunity to see the NHS at work and to gain some understanding of the pace and style of clinical practice in the UK. However, such opportunities may be difficult to access. Some hospitals make it a policy to refuse requests from overseas or refugee doctors to sit in, on the grounds that they are already overloaded with students and trainees. Others make a charge, which refugee doctors can ill afford to pay. Still others agree to let the applicant sit in on clinics but fail to make any effort to introduce or involve the doctor in any way, so that the experience is barren. We have come across refugee doctors who have felt ignored by the team they have been attached to. In some instances there has been open resentment, as supervising the refugee doctor has been perceived as an additional demand on hard-pressed time. Many report that their attachments have served no instructive purpose other than to provide a local reference based on their limited involvement. They have stuck with the attachments for this reason and also to register on their CVs their participation in a process that is becoming almost mandatory before medical employment in the UK for both overseas and refugee doctors.

In order to address these problems, and to make the clinical attachment a brief but confidence-boosting experience, we developed the concept of organising structured clinical attachments for cohorts of 5–6 refugee doctors learning together, and supporting each other, under the supervision of a tutor. Feelings of rejection and problems encountered during the attachment were explored and managed during regular group meetings with the tutor. This highly successful scheme is described in detail in Chapter 9.

PRIME Project

A new scheme is now in progress for refugee doctors who require substantial support to gain medical employment. The PRIME Project (Placing Refugee doctors In Medical Employment) is a logical development from clinical attachments as refugee doctors are placed at SHO grade in specialties of their choice for six months. This allows them to have hands-on experience instead of being observers and supervising consultants are able to evaluate the doctor's clinical abilities. Guidelines are provided to participating consultants to ensure refugee doctors are closely supervised in the first two months and are then given graduated responsibilities over the next four months according to the doctor's clinical ability. From these placements refugee doctors who are clinically competent usually manage to obtain medical jobs in open competition and continue with their medical careers.

An important lesson learned from the clinical attachment scheme is that refugee doctors require support from their peer group and from regular contact with a tutor. This was achieved by placing doctors in cohorts of 5–6 doctors in each group under the supervision of a project tutor. Feelings of rejection and problems encountered during attachments were actively managed and solved during the regular meetings of each cohort with tutors. The cohort concept has therefore been extended to the PRIME Project by placing cohorts of 8–10 doctors in SHO posts in each of two participating trusts under the supervision of a project tutor. We hope the outcome of this project will be more successful than the individual supernumerary placements that have been previously organised.

Box 2.2: Ways of helping refugee doctors back to work

- Advisory services (telephone or face to face)
- Career counselling
- Structural clinical attachments in cohorts
- Supernumerary posts
- Direct placement into established posts
- Psychological support services

Psychological support

In addition to the practical difficulties that refugee doctors face in getting back to work, there are also serious psychological challenges to be overcome. Given the appalling experiences that many of these people have survived, it is not surprising that they may demonstrate symptoms of post-traumatic stress disorder, some within the clinical threshold of illness. At the heart of all projects set up for these doctors is the need to build in a system of psychological support. In our experience these doctors usually turn down any offer of explicit psychological referral, although practical support and advice are well received and peer support is greatly appreciated. It may be that refugee doctors feel that acceptance of psychological referral might compromise their employability. Access to a reliably confidential service such as MedNet in London or House Concern in Newcastle may make such professional support more acceptable. Healthcare is stressful, even for doctors practising in their home territory and enjoying the support of friends and family. How much more so for refugee doctors, however eagerly they look forward to a return to medical work.

References

1   Hem E and Bordahl PE (2001) A 'need not possible to describe by words' – physician refugees 1939–40. *Tidsskr Nor Laegeforen.* **10**(30): 3568–73.

2   Weindling P (1998) Austrian medical refugees in Great Britain: from marginal aliens to established professionals. *Wien Klin Wochenschr.* **110**(4–5): 158–61.

3   Dubovsky H (1989) The Jewish contribution to medicine. Part III. The 19th and 20th centuries in the USA. *S Afr Med J.* **76**(3): 119–20.

4   Gonzalez A (2003) Refugee doctors. *BBC Radio 4,* 26 June.

5   Elliot P (1998) Hidden talents. *Health Service J.* **108**: 28.

6   Berlin A, Gill and Eversley J (1997) Refugee doctors in Britain: a wasted resource. *BMJ.* **325**(suppl): 262–5.

7   Linden M (2003) Posttraumatic embitterment disorder. *Psychother Psychosom.* **72**: 195–202.

8   Berlin A and Cheeroth S (2002) Clinical attachments for overseas doctors. *BMJ.* **325**(suppl): 160–1.

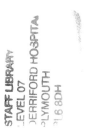

CHAPTER 3

Views and experiences of refugee doctors: a long and painful journey to start again

Dilzar Razak Kader and Zharghoona Tanin

Dr Dilzar Razak Kader

Background

I remember when I was studying back in my small town which had a population of only 20 000 I was achieving the highest scores in the primary and secondary school. My dreams started from that time to enter medical college. People were encouraging everyone who had the highest scores to study medicine. They were encouraging you to be a doctor to help poor people. I recall I was always top of my class and so I was psychologically, socially, academically and even physically a very happy boy. I entered school in the autumn of 1960 (September) and finished my primary, secondary and A levels by July 1972. To be accepted into the college of medicine in Baghdad, which was the most important college of medicine in Iraq, you had to have achieved a high score in centrally organised final exams.

I knew almost all of the people from my town and they would greet me when I was going to the school or public areas. They would congratulate me on becoming a student in the medical college

Medical school

I started to study medicine in September 1972 in Baghdad. This was a very dramatic change in my life. Previously I did all my studies at home with my family. I now had to study in a strange environment. At this time I had to face many new challenges.

I had to learn Arabic in its correct form, as the language which is used in the market or between people is colloquial and much different from that which is used in the textbooks. Often people would ask if you were Kurdish. On many occasions my friends and I had been teased for our incorrect colloquial Arabic speech.

I had to live alone and independently. I had to take care of everything myself i.e. buying my food, preparing it, washing my clothes and self-care. Previously all these things had been done for me by my family back home in Koya, my small town.

Another change was that I had to study all the subjects in English. I had to attend lectures to learn whereas before I learned only by reading books because there is an official standard of books one has to use. At first I found attending lectures in the medical college a very difficult task as in order to absorb the information as the lecturer was speaking, you had to follow him very quickly. In the first year of medical college I was only able to write down half of the lecture but this did not only apply to me and I soon found out that the majority, if not all, the students face the same problem. So we were gathering together at the end of the lecture to help each other to correct, complete, add or cancel information for our notes.

Yet another change in my life in Baghdad was that I became isolated. I needed to be alone, without distractions, to enable me to study and as this took up most of my time I did not have time to socialise. When I was back home in my small town I was studying for a few hours and at the end of the day, socialising and enjoying myself with my friends and classmates, walking and sometimes playing football.

In Baghdad I was studying most of the time in the library or in my room away from my brother who was also studying in Baghdad. He was enjoying his life. This was another psychological trauma. During the time I was studying I was feeling that I was unlike my brother and all the others. In the beginning I felt distanced from my old friends. So my first year in Baghdad University was a traumatic change in my life and I learned a lot in that year.

I also had to study until late every night. This was a new change for me because previously when I was studying for my GCSE and A levels I was studying for just a few hours.

When I passed the final exams I was very happy. I finished my University study by the end of June 1978.

Working as a doctor

When I graduated at the end of June 1978 I started to work as a doctor in Sulaymania Hospital which was one of the teaching hospitals in Iraq at that time and which was also connected to the University.

To graduate from the college of medicine and to be a doctor is also a very nice change from being a student. Now you have your own independence and a salary. You are respected amongst people. There are always people helping you in your work, for example nurses, reception and clerical staff. So you are working as a team leader. The patients, their families and people respect you. These were all positive aspects of being a doctor. At the same time I had to treat patients after official hours. which often involved working long nights but at the same time I had a lot to learn from my senior doctors and consultants. I did a full rotation in medicine, surgery, obs and gynae, paediatrics and other specialties. I finished my rotation by 1980. In Iraq you have an obligation to join the army service after finishing the rotation. So in 1980 I had to join the army to do army service.

Life in the army brought about many new changes in my life. In the army you have to be old-fashioned. The clothes you had to wear were of very poor quality. You had to wear very heavy shoes and you had to train in the sun and to start training very early in the morning – 4.00am. You were under the control of a sergeant who was usually a very ignorant man. Most of them were not able to write their names and they were ordering you to do difficult, strenuous physical army service. Unfortunately during this time the Iraq and Iran war started and we suffered a lot from this war. We also received very little money.

After we finished our time in the army we came back to the civil service again.

After this I had to do my training which included: GP training, senior house officer in paediatrics, psychiatry and general medicine. I studied DCH in Baghdad. After I finished the diploma, which lasted for a year, I came back to Arbil Children's Hospital, which is in a Kurdish area north of Iraq, and I became a lecturer in Arbil University (College of Medicine).

A lecturer and specialist paediatrician

When I finished my DCH in October 1988 I came back to Arbil Children's Hospital and I started to work as a specialist paediatrician. There were always some junior doctors with me, like house officers and senior house officers. I was in charge of the team. This was also a very positive change in my life because I became a specialist paediatrician and was respected socially, professionally and financially. I also started to teach students about paediatrics in the college of medicine in Arbil University.

I enjoyed my teaching and I was very keen to teach. I received no money from teaching. I had to teach theory to medical students. I also had to teach sessions in practical skills. I continued with this job until I came to the UK.

I was very happy with the students and I received many letters from the Deanery of the College (letters of appreciation and thanks for my service to students).

To come to the UK as a refugee

I came to the UK at the end of December 1988. When I landed in this country my aim was to work as a doctor because I had spent most of my productive life studying, practising and teaching medicine. I do believe that a doctor when he loses his profession suffers a lot because to become a doctor is not an easy thing.

As I mentioned in the background above, I can guarantee that doctors in my country are very hard-working students and have a very high IQ. They are very serious-minded people who work extremely hard. They spend the majority of their time studying and practising medicine. For this reason I feel that it would be a shame for me to leave my profession. So I asked some of my Kurdish colleagues for advice. They advised me to contact the Southwark College, as there was a famous medical English course there. I spent a few days at home organising myself and joined the course in January 1999. I contacted Sam McCarter who gave me a place on an intensive course. The courses, which are allocated for doctors to pass, are called IELTS, which is International English Language Testing System. Studying IELTS is easy but passing the exam is not easy. I have studied medicine in my country in English. However, IELTS is very different from our English. I do admit that the English we learned back home is different from the language that we use in the UK. For this reason IELTS was not an easy study. Furthermore, in order to be exempted from PLAB examination, I have to get each subject in IELTS scoring seven or more.

I did two trials at the end of which I passed IELTS and I obtained the score which was required for exemption. Meanwhile, I passed MRCPCH Part 1. I do believe that IELTS is helpful for improving a person's skills regarding English. I personally do not think it reflects the person's capability of English because there are many tricks and skills which you learn in the course.

Clinical attachment

Coming from a Kurdish town north of Iraq during the sanction time to a high standard of medical practice in the work (London) is not an easy change. For this reason I have to learn a lot. I wrote 22 letters to the hospitals in London to obtain a clinical attachment. Fortunately I received three positive responses, which were Ealing Hospital, Great Ormond Street Hospital and Northwick Park Hospital. I am thankful and grateful to all these hospitals. However, the Ealing Hospital and the Great Ormond Street Hospitals were asking for fees for clinical attachment. I think a doctor who has no job finds it very difficult to pay fees. For this reason I did not attend the interview for Great Ormond Street or Ealing Hospital. However, Northwick Park responded to my letter and accepted me for a clinical attachment (I am very grateful to them). So I started in February 2002 to do a clinical attachment in the paediatric department in Northwick Park Hospital. I found the practice of medicine in this country different to a great extent from my country.

Communication

In my country when we were prescribing prescriptions for a patient, we would explain to them briefly that they have to take these medicines for a few days and that they should come to us when they are not feeling happy. The conversation was to that extent. In this country I see communication takes a very big bulk of the doctors' time. The patient asks about the diagnosis, the treatments, the investigations and the prognosis and even about the detailed consequences of this. In this country you have to spend a lot of time talking to patients, which in my country was a very limited time. I learned a lot from the British system regarding communication.

Documentation

Although back home I was documenting the physical findings and history from the patient, the documentation was just once a day when I was seeing the patients as inpatients. The documentation did not concentrate on the feeding, psychological feelings or the general aspects of the patient. We were focusing mainly on the patient's medical problem. In this country you have to document everything, including the telephone communications.

Teamworking in this country

In my country the doctor is the leader of the team and the others have to listen to him and to follow his advice and recommendations and there is very little chance to argue with the consultant. In this country the doctors, the nurses and the therapists are all working together to offer the best service to their patients. This was also a new experience for me. For example, when I had to come down to the level of the patient (a baby who was sitting on the floor) in order to talk to him, I had to forget I am a doctor, a mature man and a professional.

The nurses play an important role in this country.

The other change in this country was the time of working. Back home I was working 8.00am–1.00pm or 8.00–2.00pm which was increased during the war, except for Thursday which ends by about 12.00. Here we have to work nine hours from nine to five and we have to come a half hour earlier. Another thing, we have no right to leave the hospital before completing everything with the patient. This was also a new change because in my country when the official time finishes you have the right to leave the hospital.

Another thing I learned in this country is that we have to work all the time and there is little chance for socialisation during the work and there is little chance to follow your personal issues while you are in the workplace. Back home we were able to receive visitors, including relatives, friends and some known patients, treating them in your spare time. Here we have no spare time and there is no time for relatives, friends and others so you may be blamed by your community for this.

Medical practice

Another change in medical practice I found here is that a doctor should work sometimes as a porter, sometimes as a domestic. For example, I have not taken any blood from patients in my country. The nurses carried this out. The nurses used to carry out cannulations. These nurses have very good relationships with the children.

I learned how to take the bloods from a patient – I had to arrange all the procedures by myself. I have also had to take the blood tests to the laboratory, sometimes by myself.

Another change, which came to me, was that I had to do night oncalls. I had not done night oncalls for a long time.

Social change

When you come to this country there is a dramatic change in the social relationships in comparison to our social relationships. Although the area seems to be safer politically, it is unsafe in other aspects. You have to take children to the school and accompany them for shopping. You have to be cautious when someone talks to you in bars, in the underground or in the shopping centres. Given all these differences, Britain is a very nice community for me and I like it. However, where we came from we had a very active social community where we knew our neighbours and the neighbours of the neighbours, which does not seem to be the case here in London. We have a lot of relatives and friends who have positive relationships with you, giving you support, sympathy, assistance and social contact. Here you have to spend most of the time alone in your home and it is very difficult to contact or communicate with people even when you know them. In other words, they have no time, no facilities or no interest.

Housing

When I came to this country there were a lot of problems regarding my social life. I lived in a flat, which was very small, and there was no space for me to read and no garden, which I have been used to back home.

I would like to express my thanks to the London Deanery, specifically Dr Michael Bannon, the groups working to help refugees like myself and all the people who were behind the scheme for refugee doctors which was a 'rescue' for many refugee doctors. I do appreciate this scheme from the bottom of my heart.

Motivation

After finishing my clinical attachment I applied for many posts as an SHO in paediatrics in different areas in the UK, including Carlisle, and applied for many posts in the East but I was not successful in gaining a position. They were using Catch 22. When I was applying for an SHO post they told me that I had too much experience for an SHO job. When I asked for a staff grade or a registrar's job they said no posts were available. At the same time they told me that in order to be a registrar or staff grade, you have to train as an SHO doctor. So Catch 22 caused a lot of problems for me, torture and anxiety. I applied for many jobs and I have been shortlisted on five or six occasions but so far have not been successful in finding a position. This obviously resulted in my becoming worried and very anxious. I started to lose hope, ambition and drive because I was told there were no vacant posts for mature doctors and very few posts for refugees. Although they claim in this country to be non-discriminating I believe this is not the case. I also believe it is very difficult for mature people to find work here in the UK.

Working in London

One day Dr Michael Bannon, Associate Dean of Postgraduate Medicine from the London Deanery, told me that there is a post for an SHO, which was regulated and run by the London Deanery. You can join this scheme which gives you a basic salary and you have to do basic hours from 9.00am to 5.00pm. When he suggested this I felt that there was hope that I would be able to become a doctor in this country again. At last I could look forward to the future and my ambitions returned. So a dramatic and positive change occurred again here in Northwick Park Hospital when Dr Bannon offered a basic salaried post to me as an SHO in Northwick Park Hospital. After doing a long clinical attachment of about six months, I became a paid doctor and an SHO in Northwick Park Hospital.

At the beginning I suffered in that I thought some of my colleagues were thinking that our practice is not as good as they would like, that our practice is different from their practice and some of them were unhappy for no apparent reason. However, there were those who were totally positive and supportive towards me. This latter group included consultants, registrars, SHOs and some nursing and clerical staff. I have now become a doctor again and am happy working in the hospital and am proud to wear my badge with my name on it. (Back home in my country no one displays their name when they are working in the hospital because people automatically know who you are.) After finishing my first six-month basic salaried job, which was paid by the London Deanery, I secured another 12-month job in Northwick Park Hospital again, thankfully.

I have to mention that in Northwick Park Hospital many people were helpful, supportive and sympathetic towards me. The permanent nursing staff in this country has a lot of experience and skills, which can help you. The other positive thing, which I found in this country, is that there is no blame policy. Here in this country it is very easy for you to tell people that you do not know and they will accept it. However, here you can ask for help from your colleagues, which is a very nice, very positive thing. They will endeavour to teach you as much as they can, so for the newcomer in this country he or she must be able to ask people for their advice and learn from it.

Summary

I found that studying, living and working in the UK is much different from the dreams I had when I was a young student in Iraq. There are many obstacles and difficulties to overcome such as cultural diversities, social communication with your working colleagues, neighbours and family, longer working hours, study time and preparation of documentation.

As work contracts are usually quite short in this country, you are changing your job and therefore you have to constantly update your CV and attend interviews. The process of finding another job is psychologically very tiring, particularly when you do not succeed in obtaining a new position and you have the added worry of not being employed whilst you are looking for a new job.

I have to travel a lot to attend courses and to attend interviews.

A positive aspect in this country is that there are many organisations, institutions and lots of good people who are able and willing to offer support to new refugee doctors. However, I do believe that you have to work harder in this country than in Iraq and that you have to be more flexible and build changes into your past medical professional experience.

Finally, you have to face a lot of changes in your life when you come to the UK. You have to be able to work as part of a team, produce clear and detailed documentation, communicate with patients and their relatives and adapt to change, be multiskilled and have an awareness of cultural diversity.

I would like to express my thanks and gratitude to all those organisations and people who enable refugee doctors and their families to meet the challenges they face in this country, regaining their confidence and being able once more to look forward to the future. Without the continuing support of these people and organisations the skills learned by many refugee doctors would have been lost for ever. However, as a result of this valuable lifeline, the doctors, their families and the British public have benefited and hopefully this will improve the service to all patients in our hospitals and surgeries.

Dr Zharghoona Tanin

Background

I have been entitled to continue my work as a doctor in the UK since August 1996. However, for five years I have been unable to work, despite applying for hundreds of posts in an atmosphere of despair and frustration. Looking back on this experience is to this day extremely difficult. In those years, all my applications for posts in obstetrics and gynaecology did not appear to make any impression on people who were supposedly aware of how their hospitals suffered from a lack of sufficient and experienced medical personnel. I was only short-listed once for an SHO post in Bristol Hospital's obstetrics and gynaecology department. However, at the end of the interview I was told that I was too senior for the job. Before I could have any glimmer of hope in finding work, I increasingly felt that perhaps the country had no need for me, that few thought that both the country and we could benefit from professionals who have come and are living in this country.

I was a consultant in obstetrics and gynaecology, medical director of the main women's hospital and a university lecturer in Afghanistan. I also worked as a doctor outside Afghanistan, in India and France. During my 13 years of medical experience I gained considerable skills and experience in obstetrics and gynaecology as well as general practice.

At the beginning of the 1990s, I was forced to leave my country with my family as all hope for peace and security in Afghanistan was lost. We went to France where we were granted asylum. There, I began to learn the French language. It was not an easy undertaking, but the organisations which were involved in the integration of refugees supported my efforts in improving my language skills as well as enabling me to receive an attachment and later a post as a part-time practitioner in the obstetrics and gynaecology department in the main hospital in the city of Tours (1994–95). I worked in the hospital until I moved to Britain where my husband, a prominent journalist, was offered a post.

In Britain, my experience in Afghanistan, India and France was taken into account. I was offered a one-year attachment and was exempt from the PLAB test on the basis of the Senior Doctor Route. This enabled me to receive a limited registration in my specialty. I started this one-year attachment in an obstetrics and gynaecology department in London. However, at the beginning of my attachment my sponsor, who was the head of the department, retired. I continued until the end without any necessary guidance, having neither mentor nor any support for my future plans and career. Subsequently, I was left with the only option of competing in a complicated jobs market, which meant applying only for certain positions, namely limited to the post of Senior House Officer. I later discovered that the situation was rather complicated: I was applying for an SHO position, whilst considered as 'overqualified', furthermore possibly seen as less suitable due to my age and my non-UK medical educational background. For the more qualified positions, passing the MRCOG examination, consisting of two parts, was necessary. I obtained Part 1 in March 1999, but was not eligible to participate in Part 2 since I did not have at least two years' work experience in the UK.

Obstacles

Limited registration meant I could apply for junior and middle-grade posts. However, I was considered too experienced for the junior posts, whilst middle-grade posts required the MRCOG Part 1 at least. It should be noted that having obtained the MRCOG Part 1 in 1999 did not alter my circumstances much. I sent hundreds of application forms containing my credentials to most hospitals throughout the country, without success. I believe that the absence of any feedback, interview and other forms of direct contact and equally a mentor or an organisation to support me made matters worse. After two years of hopeless attempts in a very competitive area I began to realise that there was something wrong either with my approach or with the system.

In retrospect, there were a number of issues that I had to pay more attention to. That of presentation was crucial in that as a doctor my qualification and experience should have been better presented. This consists of how the CV and the application statements are written, how to communicate in English and how to present one's references. Most of these have not applied to my past culture of work back in Afghanistan. Certainly this problem may apply for most refugee doctors. Recent experiences such as having an attachment or attending courses are equally impressive for people who are judging on paper. However, the most important thing is being advised or guided by a senior-level mentor whose advice and support would help to convince and change a sceptical environment to understand the merits of an experienced doctor and help them to join the health service. A senior-level mentor would also help one to keep informed of the rules and regulations and any changes that may affect one's particular situation.

Nevertheless, not everything depends on presentation or guidance. Laws and regulations and the attitude of those responsible for the employment of medical professionals (or the implementation of the employment culture) may also create impenetrable barriers.

When I was continuing to apply for a job in obstetrics and gynaecology without any success, I was told by well-intentioned medical experts that my problem was that of being in a very competitive scene because, despite the need for more gynaecology consultants, the planners did not create enough posts. They also added that the latter had no plans to provide people like me with an opportunity to be 'retrained' or absorbed in the health system. I was once advised to try to seek RCOG's help in getting a specialist training scheme. However, the final answer was that such a scheme did not exist for a refugee doctor; the training schemes were designed for national or overseas doctors. In fact, a refugee doctor was seen as neither a national nor an overseas professional.

The fixed standards of health authorities which committed themselves to safe-guarding of professional standards put people like me for years in professional abandonment. As mentioned earlier, most middle and senior posts required completion of MRCOG and sometimes also full registration, which I was unable to do without two years working in the UK. Furthermore, getting a post – obviously a junior post – was also subject to free competition based on law. Practically, in most cases a refugee doctor in a free competition post goes to the bottom of the selection. The reasons for this are obvious: when amongst tens or hundreds of applicants for one or more posts, the employer may first consider the applicant's medical educational background, their work experience, work gaps, age, sex or race which should not be considered by law. For an employer with many people in demand for a job, the 'interest' of service comes first despite the commitment of some hospitals to equal opportunity. Consequently the dynamic of free competition is less favourable for a refugee doctor, particularly those who graduated from an 'unknown' medical university, who worked in an 'unknown' hospital, whose work was disrupted by years of being uprooted and whose English is considered as a second language, etc.

Ignorance

Fixed standards and a lack of budget for employing more, much-needed medical professionals have helped some employers to stick to their own preferences. Without positive discrimination to support a balance between the interests of the employer and the interests of the country in bringing less expensive refugee professionals into the workforce, an employer could simply dismiss one's experience, no matter how good it may be, in favour of a UK-trained doctor (or an acceptable former colony-trained one) at the standard age of mid-20s.

In fact, allowing employers to bend the system one way could make discrimination and racism sometimes unavoidable. For five years, I repeatedly felt ignored, despite my experience, enthusiasm for work and my knowledge of different cultures and languages. Ignored because the system was based on an ignorance of those professionals who are seen as a burden rather than an asset for the economy; ignorance of employers who rather accommodate their own choices; ignorance of a culture which sees refugees with a black and white judgement of tabloid media and xenophobic thoughts of the extreme Right. Refugee doctors, like other refugees, have been discriminated against. The stereotype is always around: refugees are the source of unemployment, insecurity, squandering of taxpayers' money and the dissolution of British culture. But those who disseminate these stereotypes and persuade people that all or most refugees are here to make life difficult for people ignore the real contribution of thousands to the economy, prosperity, cultural and scientific richness of the country. Refugee doctors are here because they were forced to leave their country of origin. But in return they can do a lot to help a national effort build an adequate health service in this country.

New move

At the end of the 1990s the government and the health authorities recognised the urgency of the need for more doctors, nurses and medical personnel in years to come. The idea of 'importing' doctors, nurses and other medical professionals appeared to be one of the solutions. The main emphasis was on the forthcoming shortage of GPs. In the middle of the debate it appears that the authorities noticed the presence of an 'army' of refugee medical professionals, particularly doctors, who are already in the country and need few resources to be prepared to fill the gap. Now more than 850 refugee doctors are estimated to be registered with the BMA and the real figure is thought to be much more. It is now obvious how cost-effective it may be to help refugee medical professionals to meet the required standards for work and avoid wasting millions of pounds in training or 'importing' of the same number of doctors and other professionals for the health service.

Disillusioned and frustrated with the prospect of work as a doctor, in 1998 I started to approach a number of authorities in the London Deanery who were in support of the integration of refugee doctors into the health system. I wanted their advice and most importantly their help. Letters worked little. Instead it was essential to see and talk to them. Their advice and sympathy were important but not enough, particularly in cases of doctors like me who were permitted to work in their respective specialties. The lack of adequate resources and a number of rules and regulations have limited their power to deal with disadvantageous positions that most refugee doctors are in. In order to enable a refugee doctor to be absorbed into the health system they needed to have money and planning as well as the authority and power to negotiate a number of obstacles with different NHS officials and law-makers. In my case it took more than two years to be on the track and I began to work in August 2002. It became only possible with the help of the London Deanery as part of its plan and effort to overcome those obstacles that doctors in my situation faced.

A window of opportunity

With the helping hand of the health authorities, the London Deanery came up with well-defined projects for different categories of refugee doctors. In my case firstly I was put in touch with a senior consultant who agreed to act as my mentor. It was crucial for me in a situation where all my past individual efforts went nowhere to start practising my profession again. With their help I attended a series of courses designed to familiarise overseas doctors with issues such as the rules, regulations and health management in the country. I was also provided with a four-month clinical attachment at Northwick Park Hospital's paediatrics department. However, the 'preparation' period unexpectedly took about two years, for which only bad luck or bureaucracy could be held responsible.

I was first offered a six-month direct placement in an SHO post in St Mary's paediatrics department. But I lost the post as it took longer for the GMC to permit me to work in paediatrics. The London Deanery then provided me with a one-year direct placement in an SHO post in the department of obstetrics and gynaecology in Northwick Park Hospital from September 2002. It was my long-awaited return to my profession after five years of frustration and disappointment. Just before the end of this post I have secured a further SHO position at Northwick Park Hospital. I am now looking ahead trying to find how to build a new professional future.

One year of work in an SHO post in Northwick Park Hospital has some important lessons for me and for people who helped my return to work. For me, the help and guidance of the Deanery were essential. But it would have been difficult to return to work and carry out my work as a doctor effectively without having attended a series of courses, taken an attachment and finally being put in a purposeful direct placement post. During this year I have learned that in any attempt to enter in a professional competition market and start again, at least three issues are important: an overall command of English, a time for refreshing medical knowledge and practice and an opportunity to be familiarised with the UK pattern of patient management. These are not going to be achieved without having a short period followed by an opportunity of direct placement.

In my view all refugee doctors will need continuing support by the deanery until they are on stable ground from which to pursue their careers. Helping people to have a direct placement is only half the job and many refugee doctors would be in a difficult position to make a professional prospect if they are left alone. Perhaps much closer co-operation between the deanery and the health authorities would help to bring more experienced doctors into the health system to address the need for GPs and staff grades in community health services and hospitals. More positive steps in this regard would be in the real interest of the country.

CHAPTER 4

Health services in the UK

John Eversley

Introduction

The National Health Service (NHS) directly employs over 800 000 people and many more work as contractors or suppliers to it. In 2002 it spent just over £44 billion. There are many different agencies in the NHS, many services and many professions. Any detailed description is bound to be out of date very quickly. This chapter therefore only attempts to give an overview, highlighting major features and trends, with some particular observations that might be relevant to refugee doctors both in relation to their own status and development and meeting the needs of refugee patients if they have a special interest or responsibility in working with them.

Strategic decision makers

The strategic decision makers in the NHS officially are the politicians and top civil servants in the Department of Health (DH). In practice, though they may be the 'brain' of the NHS organism, they respond to signals and stimuli from outside and within the NHS. The top politician is the Secretary of State for Health. He or she is supported by a handful of more junior ministers. As well as the NHS, s/he is also responsible for planning social services, though the delivery is largely organised by social services departments of local authorities. The boundaries of the department change. Recently, responsibility for many aspects of the care of children has moved to the Department for Education and Skills (DfES) and responsibility for mental health tribunals, for example, is probably moving to the new Department for Constitutional Affairs.

The top civil servants include those with clinical and managerial backgrounds in the NHS and those with a more general management or professional background. As well as the central civil servants based in London and Leeds, England is divided into smaller areas. Currently there are 28 of these called strategic health authorities (SHAs). Officials run these but they also have non-executive members overseeing what they do. They are currently merging with the bodies responsible for planning medical and non-medical recruitment and training – the workforce development confederations.

At the national level the DH has set up a refugee health professionals steering group to oversee work on the issues. It has a number of outside people on it, advising the department.

Although the strategic decision makers are particularly responsible for the overall long-term direction of the NHS, short-term pressures that might be created by media or political interest in an issue also influence them. There are some enduring strategic issues they must address.

Even before the NHS started in 1948, there was concern about how to make the most of the available resources to meet the potential healthcare needs of the population. The overall strategy is broadly to stop the population getting seriously ill in the first place (self-care, prevention, early intervention) and if they do get ill, to treat people at home or as outpatients (primary care and community health services) and to control entry to the more expensive and specialist services (usually in hospitals). This overall strategy raises a number of challenges.

The importance of addressing wider agendas

Self-care and the prevention of ill health are very largely outside the control of the NHS. That means that the DH has to be aware of the importance of economic and social conditions (unemployment, poor working conditions and housing), attitudes and behaviour (education, alcohol, tobacco, illegal drugs). It has to convince other government departments to act on these issues to improve health and it has to demonstrate that spending on healthcare contributes to wider economic, social and political agendas. Whether refugee health professionals are encouraged to practise in the UK is exactly the kind of issue that the DH has to negotiate with other government departments.

The need to control spending on acute care

Secondly, although prevention, early intervention and treatment at home might make good sense from a public health point of view, the bulk of NHS spending (75%) is on acute care in hospitals. Successive governments have been trying to find ways of ensuring that hospitals ('secondary care') are only used when the capacity of primary care to manage illness is reached. In 1948, the main tool for doing this was by limiting direct access to hospitals by making GP referral the main route to secondary care. For a variety of reasons, this only partially worked. In the 1990s, the Conservative government introduced GP fundholding. The idea was that if GPs held the budget for hospital care, they would both do more themselves and also spend it wisely – 'commissioning' rather than using services. Since 1997, the Labour government has replaced fund-holding with primary care trusts. This is a similar idea except that community health services (nursing, therapies and social services) are involved in the commissioning.

It is likely that there will be further changes to how the commissioning of services takes place. One model is health management organisations (HMOs) acting like brokers trying to get the best deal for patients. Another model is to have very broad groups of people with an interest in healthcare, called 'stakeholders', jointly commissioning.

At the moment, the decision about whether to take positive action to recruit refugee health professionals primarily lies with the education confederations (merging with SHAs), primary care and other trusts.

Accountability

The stakeholder engagement model also reflects other challenges. On the one hand, the strategic decision makers want central control – to make sure their goals are achieved, that there is fairness in who gets services and to put things right when they go wrong. On the other hand, they cannot be (and do not want to be) responsible for day-to-day decisions. A lot of structural change in the NHS and debate takes place around 'accountability' for decisions. At the moment a government proposal for 'foundation trusts' is the focus for a lot of that discussion, with some people saying it makes accountability better and others saying it makes it worse. Presently primary care, mental health and acute trusts all have a similar structure of non-executive and executive directors who oversee the organisation. Whatever the mechanism for accountability, it is likely that many of the issues most specific to refugee doctors will only be addressed as part of wider issues such as staff recruitment and retention and service delivery equality strategies.

Also, the logic of stakeholder engagement is to decentralise decisions – to move away from central 'command and control' models. The present government initiated a set of organisational changes called 'Shifting the Balance of Power' to do this. However, the pressures of national targets and standards often act as a centralising force.

Further issues about accountability are discussed below in relation to regulation and quality.

Policy advisers/research bodies

The role of Parliamentary bodies is discussed below. Outside government and the NHS, there are a variety of bodies that analyse, advise or recommend policies and practice. They may be research bodies (including universities), consultancies, lobbyists and pressure groups.

In relation to health, and specifically refugees, the King's Fund is important. It is a charitable body that does research, gives grants (not to individuals) and facilitates policy discussions. It has supported work both on the health needs of refugee communities and on recognition of refugee health professionals. The Wellcome Trust is a similar organisation supporting more clinical research and work on history that has included work on refugee doctors.

There are a number of bodies specifically concerned with policy and research on refugees including, for example, the Refugee Council and the Information Centre About Refugees (ICAR). There are a number of bodies specifically concerned with refugee doctors. They are often non-governmental organisations (NGOs) or voluntary organisations. They include the World University Service Refugee Education and Training and Advice Service (RETAS) and the Jewish Council for Racial Equality (JCORE). Many of these bodies come together with professional and educational bodies in the British Medical Association's Refugee Doctors Group.

Perhaps the real challenge for refugee doctors is to ensure that their concerns are reflected in the work of the more general think-tanks and consultancies concerned with health and public policy and management that have not taken up the specific issues. There are many of them and their names are to be found in the broadsheet newspapers and the journals concerned with public services.

Funding

Almost all NHS funding for running costs (revenue) comes from the Treasury and is paid for by taxation. The relatively small amount of money that comes from NHS charges does not add to NHS resources and money from the NHS selling services privately is insignificant. Revenue is allocated to SHAs which in turn allocate it to primary care trusts and other trusts. The allocation to SHAs is based on a formula that takes into account the size and needs of the population and the costs of providing services. The primary care trusts use some of the money to buy services from other trusts. Money for general practice comes through formulae that are negotiated nationally (General Medical Services – recently changed significantly) or locally (Personal Medical Services). There has been much criticism of the allocation formulae for not adequately reflecting the needs of refugee communities.

Although most Treasury money comes in block grant to the DH, there is some money that can be bid for to fund schemes that spend money to save money, for example 'Invest to Save'. A small scheme to support refugee doctors has already been successful. A larger proposal is planned.

The way that money for buildings and major items of equipment (such as computer systems) is arranged is more complex. The government believes the money has to come from the private sector and is promoting the Private Finance Initiative (PFI) to do this generally and for primary care a scheme called LIFT. In both cases it generally involves the private sector building or buying capital and managing it on behalf of the NHS.

Service planning

Trying to spend the NHS's money and use its resources effectively takes a lot of planning. The names of the plans and the bodies that do the planning are constantly changing but the types of plan are broadly the same.

The government has overall plans for spending and services. The DoH usually has one overall grand plan that is meant to cover a long period (often 10 years). Currently, it is called the NHS Plan. Overall statements of government policy are generally called White Papers. When a plan is proposed for consultation, it is called a Green Paper. Often major plans require legal changes that are set out in Bills that become Acts after a Parliamentary process. Acts are often quite general and need to be supported by detailed rules or explanations that are set out in Statutory Instruments or Orders. For example, the rules regarding fitness to practise of overseas-qualified doctors are part of an Order.

Within the overall grand design there are service and spending plans at the national and local level. They are both overall plans and plans for particular sectors of healthcare. Sometimes, they are medium-term plans (3–5 years) and always there are annual plans. Governments have been trying to move away from basing plans simply on whatever was done last year (plus or minus a bit). There are many examples of trying to plan services and spending on the basis of the kind of outcome planners want to achieve expressed in terms of health status ('halving the incidence of lung cancer in 10 years'), a pattern of service ('a specialist cancer service in reach of everybody') or a workforce ('only specialist trained nurses working with children'). At the moment National Service Frameworks – for example for cancer and mental health or the White Paper on services for people with learning difficulties, called *Valuing People* – are examples of such plans. Refugees either as service providers or service users are rarely substantially considered in such plans. The challenge for refugee doctors is both to have the issues included in the first place and to demonstrate how the targets can be achieved by consideration of refugees as service users and/or providers.

Among the major areas of illness covered by the plans are cancers, coronary heart disease, diabetes and mental health. Among population groups, children, older people and people with learning difficulties and teenage pregnancies are the subject of national plans. Strategic health authorities and trusts have plans for these topics but sometimes for other disease areas or population groups.

The present government has been particularly keen on setting measurable targets for public services to achieve and recording performance. It is keen on establishing a system in which well-performing service providers are given more freedom and more money to plan how to achieve their targets. This and its implications are considered further below.

Service providers

The basic division of health services into primary, secondary and tertiary has already been referred to. The idea of a tripartite structure for the state health service in the UK goes back to the 1920s, but the boundaries and content of each part have evolved.

Primary care

'Primary care' in many developing countries (following World Health Organization definitions) is more broadly construed than in the UK. The development of healthy living centres (often funded through the National Lottery) or health promotion activities targeted at particular groups reflects this wider conception. Sometimes in the UK the term is used very narrowly to mean only general medical practice. More usually, it includes the four family health services (FHS) – general medical and dental practice, optometry (dispensing opticians) and pharmacists (high-street chemists) and some community health services (CHS: described further below). The four FHS have historically been provided by private contractors receiving fees from the NHS for providing services to NHS patients. Dentists, optometrists and pharmacists have been getting increasing proportions of their income from charging patients directly as NHS support for their services has been withdrawn. Pharmacy, dentistry and optometry are also increasingly provided through chains – Boots pharmacies, Whitecross Dental Care, Specsavers. Some people see the beginnings of a similar trend in general practice (e.g. Medicentres). About 25% of general dental practices no longer accept NHS patients, particularly adults. In some areas, community dental services run by NHS salaried dentists provide significant services to 'vulnerable groups', including refugees.

In the 1940s most GPs were strongly opposed to becoming salaried doctors and so worked under contract. The GPs who are partners in such practices are called principals. They sometimes employ assistants. Many people starting in general practice, either through choice or necessity, begin as assistants. In recent years a number of schemes (including Personal Medical Services (PMS)) have increased the number of GPs who are paid salaries by primary care trusts. About one-third of all GPs are now on PMS contracts. PMS practices sometimes target particular populations who find it hard to register with other practices, including refugees.

When the NHS was created in 1948, many community health services were run by local authorities (councils). These included district nurses (mainly working with older and disabled people), health visitors (mainly working with mothers and children), school nurses and occupational therapists. In 1974, they transferred to the NHS. Now most work for primary care trusts. There are debates about the role of all the professions with moves to emphasise the public health role of community nurses and the promotion of 'independent living' by therapists and nurses.

Access to primary care

Problems with securing access to primary care (also hospital services) have given rise to a number of types of post for people to act as intermediaries between clinicians and service users, addressing issues of language, culture and provider/ user relationships. These posts are variously called advocates, link workers, interpreters, outreach or development workers. They are often targeted at specific communities – including refugee communities – and have been a source of employment for refugee health professionals. They can be a source of familiarisation with the NHS.

Emergency care

Emergency and out-of-hours care crosses the boundaries between primary and secondary provision. Hospitals run accident and emergency (A&E) departments. However, it has been recognised for many years that many people use A&E services because of difficulty accessing GP services, especially in the evenings and at weekends ('out-of-hours'). A range of other services has emerged such as walk-in centres, NHS Direct (a nurse-led telephone and Internet-based service) and GP out-of-hours co-operatives, often based in hospitals. Emergency services for people with mental health problems or in cases of child protection can be accessed through these services, through social services departments or through the police.

Some time ago ambulance services were split into patient transport services, for outpatients and discharged patients, and the emergency ambulances. Trained paramedics now generally staff the emergency ambulance services. Fire-fighters and increasing numbers of police officers are also receiving paramedic training.

Long-term care

Local authorities historically provided long-term care for older people and disabled people in residential homes or at home. The NHS provided long-term care for people with mental health problems or learning difficulties in long-stay hospitals. Moves to replace long-stay hospitals and residential homes were called 'Care in the Community'. Since the 1980s private and voluntary services have largely replaced NHS and council provision, often in people's own homes or smaller units. Refugee health professionals have sometimes found jobs as care assistants in such services. Currently further changes are under way in how support in people's homes is being provided, with grants being paid to particular landlords to provide services 'Supporting People'. Refugees with mental health problems or physical impairments may be eligible for this kind of provision.

People with long-term or cyclical health problems may need services that span the primary/secondary/tertiary agencies: intermediate care services and outreach or satellite services often do this. Provision for people with chronic or terminal illness ('palliative care') is provided by the NHS by primary care trusts and specialist units (for cancer and AIDS patients, for example) but significant provision is by voluntary organisations. The Macmillan and Marie Curie charities, for instance, provide support to cancer patients. There are also a number of hospices providing residential and domiciliary services. Many of the hospices are run by Christian organisations, but they welcome patients of other faiths and do not evangelise or require Christian observance.

Public health

Public health has increasingly been devolved to primary care trusts. Public health jobs are also being opened up to people without recognised clinical qualifications. The work of public health or health improvement departments includes population needs assessment or profiling, infectious disease control and service reviews. Local authorities are responsible for many other public health functions such as housing conditions and hygiene in shops and eating places. Various bodies such as the Health and Safety Executive (HSE) are responsible for workplaces.

Mental health services

Mental health services also cross the primary/secondary/tertiary, health/housing and social care divides. They are increasingly provided or co-ordinated through specialist mental health trusts covering large areas. Their services generally include community mental health teams (including nursing and social care and sometimes other services, drugs and alcohol services, clinics for 'talking therapies' and counselling, pharmacological treatments for both out- and inpatients). Their specialist ('tertiary') provision includes secure provision for people who might be a risk to themselves or others and offenders. They sometimes support specialist provision such as the Medical Campaign for the Victims of Torture or the Refugee Therapy Centre.

Secondary and tertiary services

The services run by hospitals (except for accident and emergency services, sexual health services and a few others) are normally accessed via primary care. Partly because of the different histories of particular hospitals, there are big differences in the size and the range of services provided by various hospitals. Individual hospitals may be grouped together into a larger trust, e.g. Barts, the London Chest and the Royal London together make up the Barts and the London Trust. In general, the bigger trusts and more specialist trusts have a bigger role in training and research. The bigger trusts may also have more extensive diagnostic and laboratory services that may be a source of non-clinical opportunities for refugee health professionals.

What a trust does depends partly on what primary care trusts and SHAs pay for, but also on what funds it gets for training and research. The influences on training are discussed below. Government may fund research directly or through research councils. Research may also be funded by the private sector (especially pharmaceutical companies), specialist research charities such as Cancer Research UK or more general ones like Wellcome or Nuffield. Sometimes researchers themselves, the funders or the ethics committees that have to approve research make a particular point about whether the research is relevant to particular communities.

Maternity services are sometimes provided in hospital trusts and sometimes in primary care trusts. New kinds of trusts bringing together education, social and health services for children are being set up in some areas. Sometimes a specialist trust will provide services on the premises of another trust. For example, Moorfields Eye Hospital, based in north-east London, provides services to a trust in south London. Some people see the future of hospitals as more of this, like a street market or food mall where different providers both compete and collaborate.

Regulation, control and quality

One of the areas of public services where most change is taking place is how their performance is measured, by whom, strategies for improving it and what happens when things go wrong. Change is so rapid that trying to name individual agencies and their roles could only lead to inaccuracies, so this section will set out some of the general features of the system in terms of the different kinds of accountability the arrangements are intended to address. The different kinds of accountability overlap and so does the work of the agencies responsible for them.

Political accountability

Ultimately the NHS is accountable to Parliament. Ministers have to answer questions from MPs and peers. There is also a committee of MPs scrutinising health – the House of Commons Select Committee on Health. Recently, for example, it has inquired into maternity services and foundation hospitals. Individual complaints to MPs about health services can be handled by the Health Service Ombudsman. Certain aspects of the NHS are also scrutinised by the National Audit Office, which is also accountable to Parliament.

At the local level, local authorities are expected to set up health scrutiny panels or committees (not all have done so yet). These panels generally have some locally elected councillors, but also co-opted members of the public and expert advisers. In London, the Greater London Assembly has a health scrutiny committee. It has recently looked at GP recruitment and retention and its report strongly recommended more efforts to recruit refugee doctors.

Legal accountability

Legal accountability is often overlooked when considering the NHS, but the NHS is generally subject to the same laws as other employers and public services providers. If they are alleged to have broken the law, NHS bodies can face courts and tribunals.

- If an NHS body acts 'unreasonably' or not in accordance with its rules, it can be subject to judicial review.
- If the NHS breaches Health and Safety at Work legislation or its responsibility to the public or human rights legislation (including, but not only, race, sex and disability discrimination), there are remedies.
- If 'medical negligence' is alleged, a victim or relative can take civil action against the NHS.
- If an NHS employer discriminates in relation to race, sex or disability, it can be taken to an industrial tribunal. Some refugees are covered by race discrimination legislation, others are not.
- If something goes catastrophically wrong, the government sets up a judicial inquiry, such as those in the Harold Shipman or the Bristol Heart Hospital cases.

In all these situations there are professional and managerial arrangements for supporting the NHS and in most cases there are arrangements for supporting the employee or member of the public.

Managerial accountability

Within the NHS all its employees and contractors have individuals or bodies to which they are accountable. There are several distinct forms of managerial accountability.

- *Day-to-day management and supervision.* This is increasingly done through agreed work programmes for individuals and departments that may or may not be regularly reviewed. This kind of management is least practised in relation to doctors, especially GPs.
- *Internal performance management.* NHS trusts, in particular, have systems for setting, recording and improving performance. They will also have systems for managers to deal with complaints about staff from within the organisation or from the public. Responsibility for internal performance management in trusts usually rests ultimately with the board composed of the executive and non-executive directors. The new GP GMS Contract means that practice partnerships are likely to have this responsibility.
- *External performance monitoring and management.* This is the area where most change is taking place. In general, governments have been arguing that operational decisions (what to do, how to do it, how much time and money to spend) should be devolved as closely as possible to the point of service delivery. In place of central instructions, they have brought in systems of targets, monitoring and rewards and punishments for success or failure. Thus, trusts are given targets for waiting times for operations or cancelled operations. The achievement of targets is reported annually (currently on a system of nought to three stars). The management of 'no' or low-star trusts is put under intense pressure and greater control than one with three stars. The inspection agencies also conduct thematic or agency-based inspections when they visit trusts and examine all or part of its work in depth. GP practices are not yet generally or formally assessed in this way but there are moves towards it. There are many different bodies involved in external performance monitoring and there are moves to co-ordinate or merge some of them. Currently the Commission for Healthcare Audit and Inspection (CHAI) and the Audit Commission are two of the most important.

    In addition to this inspection regime, NHS agencies are given instructions and guidance. Guidance from the DoH itself usually comes in the form of Circulars or Letters. There are also a variety of NHS agencies that issue advice or instructions on a wide range of subjects such as the prescribing of drugs and the use of medical devices and equipment. Practices receive some advice and instructions of this kind.

Probably inevitably, the managerial (and financial) accountability system tends to accept the familiar and be more cautious (and sometimes hostile) to new or exceptional arrangements. This can mean that schemes for refugee populations or professionals are not recognised in performance management (and therefore 'don't count') or are subject to additional or different scrutiny.

Financial accountability

In general, all resources in the NHS are allocated for a purpose and have to be spent according to certain rules to avoid corruption and ensure 'value for money'. As well as making sure that the sums are done correctly and that the money has been spent on what it should be, this means making sure it is spent wisely – 'resource accounting'. The system is very similar (but often separate) to the system for managerial accountability.

- Day-to-day financial control by finance departments and authority delegated to departments.
- Internal audit (within finance departments).
- External audit. There is a government service, called the District Audit Service, that contracts out many of its inspections to private auditors.
- External assessment. Major plans, particularly for capital spending, normally go through a process of external approval by the Civil Service or outside experts.

Professional accountability

Historically the professions have regulated themselves individually. In recent years there has been external pressure and professional recognition of the need to include more lay people in professional regulation. As interprofessional teams and newer professions have developed, the need for collaboration between professional bodies has been recognised. As with other kinds of accountability, different bodies are responsible for different levels of accountability.

- Ultimate professional responsibility for deciding who is a professional and for professional conduct lies with the appropriate regulatory body – the General

Medical Council, Nursing and Midwifery Council, etc. They in turn are governed by legislation, mainly British but also international legislation on free movement of labour and human rights, for example.

- Standards for training and practice in each specialty within medicine are broadly set by the Royal Colleges (Surgeons, Physicians, General Practitioners).
- Within every institution there is a clinician (not necessarily a doctor) who is responsible for setting and monitoring standards and professional working arrangements – this is called 'clinical governance'.
- Within teams, there will generally be a structure of responsibility for training and supervision of junior staff and staff in training. In general medical practice, this is really limited to supervision of assistants, registrars and students.

All refugee doctors will be aware of the importance of the General Medical Council. Once they have overcome the hurdle of initial recognition, the Royal Colleges, clinical governance and senior clinicians will have an important influence on their career opportunities.

Public accountability

In theory, health services are accountable to the public, as actual or potential service users, as taxpayers or voters. The theory is not always practised.

The cornerstone of accountability to patients should be 'informed consent'. There is possibly a stronger tradition of involving patients in decisions in the UK than in some other medical cultures but it is still sometimes neglected. This is the case particularly for speakers of English as an Additional Language or people who are perceived as having impaired capacity to make decisions through mental ill health or learning disability. Refugee patients may be vulnerable to this problem.

All NHS services are required to have arrangements for hearing complaints locally and for appeal mechanisms if they are not immediately resolved. There are also arrangements for advice and liaison between patients and service providers (PALS services). Arrangements for support to patients wishing to make a complaint are currently changing. The bodies previously responsible – community health councils (CHCs) – are being abolished.

There are various national and local programmes to involve patients in other ways – deciding service priorities or assessing the quality of services, for example. There is recognition that refugees and other groups are often left out of such activities and there are initiatives to combat this.

As well as the formal structures of accountability to the public, there is no doubt that media interest – from a letter in the local newspaper through to reporting of in-depth inquiries – is influential.

Training and recruitment

Professional education for the NHS is generally provided through the universities and professional bodies such as the Royal Colleges. The system for paying for it and designing it is more complicated. The main agencies that fund and commission postgraduate training are the deaneries (for doctors) and the workforce development confederations (WDCs) for NHS staff generally. The WDCs are currently merging with strategic health authorities. Each deanery and WDC has someone responsible for international recruitment who is sometimes (but not always) also specifically responsible for refugee health professionals. Overall, however, the preoccupations of the planners, funders and providers of training are with people who have trained in the UK and are currently practising or who might return to practice. Some of the agencies need persuading that there are enough refugee health professionals who can cost-effectively be supported to recognition. There are also issues about which funds within and between agencies should be used to train refugee health professionals.

Another issue for training bodies is how much training students generally get to meet the needs of refugee communities. Responsibility for training to meet the needs of diverse populations is usually expressed quite generally. Even where training planners, funders or providers are willing to be more specific, they do not necessarily have the expertise. Some refugee health professionals have been able to provide that expertise as visiting lecturers, for example.

Recruitment to jobs in the NHS generally takes place at the level of individual institutions and most of the time they advertise externally in newspapers (national newspapers such as *The Guardian* on Wednesdays and local newspapers) and in journals. There are professional journals such as the *BMJ*, professional magazines such as *Pulse* and management magazines such as the *Health Service Journal*.

Agency staff often fill temporary jobs. The NHS has its own temporary recruitment agency – NHS Professionals – but it also uses private agencies, of which there are many. They can be found in the Yellow Pages phone directory under 'Recruitment' or 'Employment' agencies and they often have branches in or near hospitals. Private care providers use them too, particularly for providing home care.

Employee/professional bodies

In navigating round the NHS, either for oneself or on behalf of patients, refugee doctors are likely to need the support of employee and professional bodies.

Nearly all recognised, practising doctors are members of the British Medical Association. Their ambivalence historically about refugee doctors (*see* Chapter 1) has been replaced by an unambiguous commitment. The different things that they do are noted elsewhere. The Royal Colleges have generally been less organised and consistent in their support. However, the Royal College of General Practitioners has been of particular support and has had a number of leaders from refugee backgrounds.

Particularly for doctors working in non-clinical roles, trade union support may be useful. The largest health union is UNISON. In trusts, the unions (including the BMA) usually come together in a joint body to negotiate with employers, called staff side, that is part of a formal negotiating arrangement in the NHS. The staff side often has an officer responsible for equalities who may be of particular use. The staff side chair or secretary should also be accessible.

In principle, the professional bodies and trade unions will also take up issues relating to refugee communities as well as employees. UNISON has a particular record of helping people fighting deportations.

Healthcare outside the NHS

The NHS provides most healthcare in the UK. Some other types of care have already been noted. In summary, they include:

- care in the home and nursing homes provided by private and voluntary agencies
- voluntary organisations providing specialist treatment or support, e.g. palliative care, drugs and alcohol projects or mental health services
- health promotion or ill health prevention services, often working with the NHS, such as healthy living centres
- a few private hospitals and clinics and even fewer private general practices
- in the past, the prison service and armed forces had separate health services. They are increasingly integrated though the armed forces still have an entirely separate service as well as the integrated system.

In general private and voluntary provision is covered by the same professional regulation as the NHS.

Resources

- BMA: web.bma.org.uk/ap.nsf/Content/_Home_Public
- DH: www.dh.gov.uk
- Health resources for refugees: www.harpweb.org.uk
- ICAR: www.icar.org.uk
- Iles V (1997) *Really Managing Health Care*. Open University Press, Buckingham.

- In particular to keep up with changing structures in the NHS go to www.dh.gov.uk/Site Map/AboutUsMap/fs/en
- JCORE: www.re.leonet.co.uk/jcore.html
- Kings Fund: www.kingsfund.org.uk
- Klein R (2001) *The New Politics of the NHS* (4e) Prentice Hall, Harlow, Essex.
- Refugee Council: www.refugeecouncil.org.uk
- RETAS: www.wusuk.org/RETAS/retas_content.htm
- Wellcome: www.wellcome.ac.uk

CHAPTER 5

The social welfare system in the UK

John Eversley

Introduction

The system of social welfare in the UK is highly developed. About two-thirds of public spending (expected to be £257 billion out of £380 billion in 2002–03) goes on health, education and welfare. Describing the system for refugee doctors is challenging because of its size and complexity, but also because the system which they or their families or refugee patients may have to use is often not the same as the mainstream system.

Conventionally descriptions of social welfare systems are 'institutional', explaining the roles, functions and rules of all the different agencies and departments. This will not be the approach here for reasons of space and because the institutional arrangements do not necessarily reflect the way that people think of their lives. Instead, eight major categories of people's lives are identified and broad overviews of each are given.

Home life

Most people in Britain are owner-occupiers; they live in self-contained dwellings that they have bought, usually with the help of a long-term loan from a building society or bank. About a third of the population are tenants of a social landlord. This used mainly to mean local authorities (being a 'council tenant') but increasingly councils are transferring their stock to other landlords. These are mostly registered social landlords (RSLs), usually housing associations. They are not-for-profit organisations, but they have to act commercially over rent levels, arrears and repairs. Some people live in private rented accommodation. Homeless people generally live in hostels (especially if they are single) or bed and breakfast hotels (if they have children). All local authorities have homeless persons units – usually part of the housing department. Access to council housing used generally to be through a 'points' system of allocation: the more needs you had, the more points you got and, in theory, the quicker you were rehoused. Increasingly the system is changing to a 'lettings' system in which you still have to be eligible, but vacant properties are advertised and then let to the household with most needs for whom the dwelling is appropriate.

Social tenants are entitled to help with repairs. Owner-occupiers may be entitled to help with improvements (to help with heat insulation or basic amenities such as having an inside toilet). Disabled tenants and owner-occupiers may be entitled to adaptations to their home.

People on low incomes (including unemployed people and many pensioners) are entitled to help with housing costs – including council tax. This is part of a much wider system of 'social security'. Essentially the social security system has three parts to it:

- *a universal system* that entitles everybody in certain categories to cash benefits, such as Child Benefit and the state pension
- *a tax and tax credit system* that gives allowances and credits for certain costs or expenditure, such as having children
- *a selective cash benefits system* for people on low incomes or with higher living or working costs, including older people, single parents, disabled people and children.

The National Asylum Support Service (NASS) is responsible for providing both dwellings and financial support for asylum seekers. Asylum seekers may be put in bed and breakfast accommodation, hostels, detention or removal centres (including sometimes prisons or police stations).

If noisy or hostile neighbours are bothering someone, landlords, local authorities and the police should all have arrangements in place to deal with it.

None of these entitlements are straightforward and specialist housing advice services, law centres, citizens' advice bureaux or other advice agencies may be useful. GPs are often asked for help with housing problems. Although confirmation that someone has health problems and/or that poor housing is contributing is often necessary, it is not usually enough to get housing improved or changed.

Learning

Schooling is compulsory between the ages of five and 16 in the UK.

Provision for the under-fives is a mixture of private, voluntary and statutory provision. Some of it is targeted at children who are seen as vulnerable and is subsidised or free (day nurseries). Preparation for school, usually for children who are 3–4 years old (state nursery classes or schools), is also free. There are Child Tax Credits for many parents who are paying for childcare by 'approved' providers, which can include registered childminders, nurseries, crèches and playgroups.

Most 5–11-year olds go to primary (infant and junior) schools. Most are state schools run by local education authorities (LEAs). Faith groups – mostly Church of England and Catholic, but also other Christian, Jewish and Muslim communities – run some primary schools. While at primary school children will sit three sets of national tests (SATS). The tests for 11-year olds (Key Stage III) are often used as the basis of selection for secondary schools. Some LEAs and schools have separate selection tests.

In some areas, there are infants schools, middle schools and upper schools. Most 11–16-year olds go to state or state-aided secondary schools with some going to private or faith schools. There is a wider variety of secondary schools than there used to be. The system is not easy to understand. State-aided education is free, but in many schools uniforms, trips and other 'extras' have to be paid for, though help is often available. At primary and secondary schools, school lunches are provided and they are free to parents on income support. Every LEA has to publish a guide to arrangements for transfer to secondary school that explains the local situation. They also have to provide an advice service for parents. At 16, most children do public exams, called GCSEs.

At 16 children can leave school. Those who want to stay in education may go to a sixth form centre, further education or community college. Sixth forms and centres tend to concentrate on academic qualifications (AS and A levels). Further education (FE) and community colleges offer academic and more vocational qualifications. The financial arrangements for post-16 education are complicated but broadly, many students can get allowances and parents can go on claiming Child Benefit for 16–18-year olds in education.

Disabled children or children with special educational needs (SEN) may go to ordinary (mainstream or inclusive) schools or to special (separate) schools. If the children need extra or different support they are likely to have to go through an assessment process called 'statementing'.

After further education about 35% of young people go on to university. The financial arrangments for university are changing and the length of time that a young person has lived in the country or a particular area may determine how much they have to pay in fees and whether they will get an allowance of any kind. Most students depend on student loans that they are expected to repay when they start earning. Many students need to find paid work while they are studying.

There are opportunities for adults to return to study for academic or vocational qualifications or leisure interests. 'Community education' is usually organised by LEAs or by leisure departments of local authorities. Opportunities to learn English may be organised by community education, FE colleges, universities, and private language schools. Financial support is sometimes available. Particularly for people who need English for professional purposes, for example who may have to sit the IELTS tests, it is important to find courses appropriate to their needs.

Employment

For people eligible to work in the UK, there are a variety of services to help while unemployed, to find jobs and to get training. Such people may also get Job Seekers Allowance (JSA) providing they demonstrate that they are actively seeking work. For the first six months the amount of JSA is based on National Insurance contributions; thereafter it is based on income and assessed needs. While unemployed, people can do a limited amount of voluntary work. Centres, currently called Job Centre Plus, have details of some vacancies and where to get support with preparing applications, CVs and interviews, etc. Jobcentre Plus and the Pension Service are the new organisations that have replaced the Benefits Agency and the Employment Service and are part of the Department for Work and Pensions.

Much of the funding for training comes through a national network of learning and skills councils. There are specialist advisers and agencies for disabled people. For disabled people, young people, over-25s who have been out of work over 18 months, single parents, over-50s, partners of people out of work more than six months and older people, there are other specific initiatives called New Deals.

Once in employment, employers and employees have a wide range of rights and obligations. These include payment of tax and National Insurance contributions, minimum wage rates, safe working arrangements, paid holidays, sick pay arrangements, protection from discrimination, maternity and paternity leave. If in doubt about obligations or rights, individuals should contact law centres, citizens' advice bureaux, trade unions or other advice agencies.

Health and safety

An outline of the workings of the NHS is given in Chapter 4. A more detailed description of services to dispersed asylum seekers is given in the Refugee Council/ DH resource pack available at www.doh.gov.uk/asylumseekers. This section therefore focuses on community safety – the police, courts and penal system.

There is no general national police force in the UK, though there are specialist national units. Policing in London, for instance, is divided between the Metropolitan Police and the City of London Police. Traffic wardens are generally employed or contracted by local authorities – except on Red Routes!

The law is divided between civil and criminal law. Parking offences or disputes between buyers and sellers of goods and services are generally civil offences. Divorce is a civil matter. Child welfare may be a civil matter but child protection is a criminal matter. The higher courts separate out the two kinds of offences but the lower (magistrates and county) courts can hear both kinds of case. Lawyers are divided into solicitors and barristers. Although some solicitors can represent clients in the higher courts, mostly this is done by barristers. Those barristers who prosecute on behalf of the state are called Queen's Counsel (QCs). Solicitors who prosecute on behalf of the state generally work for the Crown Prosecution Service (some work for other agencies).

Magistrates are mostly unpaid lay volunteers though there are some paid ('stipendiary') magistrates. They can fine people, impose community service orders, put people on probation (behave or be punished) or send them to prison for short periods. Magistrates and county courts do not have juries. Crown courts have juries, as do some higher courts.

Except for very specialist judges, in financial cases for example, all judges are or were lawyers, mostly barristers.

Alongside the courts system is the tribunal system. Tribunals are mainly to make sure that public or administrative law is being correctly applied. There are many different kinds of tribunals including employment, mental health and immigration. Tribunal members may include lawyers but lay people are also members.

There are various specialist services to help courts make decisions. In cases involving the welfare or protection of children, there are Child and Family Court Advisory and Support Services (CAFCASS) and children can have separate support from their parents from social workers. If an expert witness is needed in a case, currently they have to appear either for the prosecution or the defence though their evidence may not be contested. Before passing sentence, judges and magistrates can order social inquiry reports. Probation officers collect information, including sometimes from doctors, about a person's background.

Another part of the judicial system is the coroner's court. The coroner (usually a lawyer or a doctor) has to determine the cause of death and they can make observations or recommendations. They may sit with a jury. Coroner's courts are likely to be radically overhauled in the near future.

The prisons service mostly runs prisons though private firms run some. Prisons and prisoners are categorised by the degree of security they need. High-risk prisoners – Category A – go to high-security prisons such as Belmarsh in south-east London. Category D prisoners may be in open prisons from which they may go out to supervised work during the day or have home leave. The prison population is considerably larger than the official capacity of the prisons and this is causing a number of problems.

For young people, there is a separate system of justice to that of adults. The Youth Justice Board oversees it and each area has a youth offending team (YOT:

joint local authority, police and probation teams) and special magistrates courts. Young people are not supposed to be sent to adult prisons, though it sometimes happens. There are young offenders institutions, for example Feltham in south-west London.

For the most common kinds of low-level crime – vandalism, car and mobile phone theft, burglary, shoplifting – in effect most of the responsibility for prevention and detection lies with the property owners. Local authorities, retailers and hospitals increasingly use closed circuit TV (CCTV) and security guards to protect property. Local authorities may also employ neighbourhood wardens to prevent problems or intervene. They may also have special antisocial behaviour teams or tenant support teams to deal with problems on estates.

Rape and domestic violence are increasingly dealt with by specialist teams of police officers (often women) working with social and health services. Counselling and safe houses (refuges) exist in many areas.

Leisure and shopping

Access to opportunities for sport, recreation and goods and services required for health, cultural or religious needs are part of the broader social welfare system. Sports facilities are often provided for or by local authorities. There are charges that may be reduced or waived for people on low incomes or who are disabled. Some health services and leisure providers collaborate to provide 'Prescriptions for exercise'. There are also many private and voluntary sports facilities and clubs. They are generally listed in Yellow Pages or Thomsons directories.

Food to meet specific dietary needs – diabetic, vegetarian, halal and kosher, for example – is generally available. There can be problems about lack of clear labelling of food – particularly additives and whether genetically modified products are included. Information for diabetics is provided by Diabetes UK and religious and ethnic organisations often provide directories about sources of appropriate food. A lot of vegetarian food is marked with a green 'V' symbol. If there are questions about the quality or content of foods, nationally, the Food Standards Agency is responsible. Local authorities also have trading standards departments responsible for inspection.

Trading standards departments are also locally responsible for questions about substandard goods or services or goods that are not what they say they are (counterfeit). Their resources and powers are, however, limited. The Consumers Association (a voluntary organisation) and National Consumers Council (a statutory body) also take up such issues.

Many public services are now run privately (gas, electricity, water, telecommunications) or by arms-length public bodies (the Royal Mail). Regulators who are supposed to control and monitor the quality and prices of services oversee them all. The titles of the regulators generally begin with 'Office of . . .', leading to OFWAT, OFTEL, OFGEM, etc. These have statutory powers. There are also voluntary trade or professional associations covering builders, solicitors, estate agents, garages, etc. They are often seen as not every effective. A government-appointed ombudsman also oversees solicitors.

The environment

The physical environment and transport are also important to health and well-being. Poorer people and new arrivals are among those most vulnerable to pollution, hazards and exclusion from travel because of cost or where they live.

Nationally the main government agency formally responsible for the quality of the physical environment is the Environment Agency. At the local level, planning and environmental health departments are responsible for setting and enforcing standards within national guidelines. As well as statutory bodies, there are many non-governmental bodies concerned with the environment, including Friends of the Earth, Greenpeace and, at the local level, many civic societies.

Public transport (trains, buses, tubes and taxis) is run by a variety of international, national and local organisations. They are generally private companies overseen by public regulators. Some transport is provided by voluntary organisations such as Dial-a-Ride schemes – mainly for older and disabled people – and community transport schemes, which sometimes run patient transport schemes.

To drive a private car in the UK you need a valid (UK or international) driving licence, an insured, roadworthy vehicle (vehicles over three years old need an MOT test but that doesn't mean they are roadworthy). To get a UK driving licence you need to pass a theoretical and a practical test. The theory test requires a reasonable level of English.

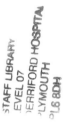

Identity and culture, personal relationships

Denial of the opportunity to practise one's religion, political or cultural beliefs or lifestyle is one reason why refugees have to leave their countries of origin. It is not always straightforward here either. Although all the major religious faiths are practised in the UK, it can be difficult to find places to worship, leaders of worship or religious teachers. There are various bodies that may help. Christian churches come together in local, national and world councils of churches and they will often help non-Christian faiths. Councils of mosques exist in many areas. All local education authorities have advisory committees on religious education (SACREs). Local councils on racial equality may be able to help with issues around ethnicity, particularly discrimination, as may the National Commission for Racial Equality. As well as specific voluntary organisations concerned with refugees, there are many other voluntary organisations. They often come together in local forums such as councils of voluntary service. All these bodies may be listed in the community pages of Yellow Pages or Thomsons directories or in libraries or on local authority websites.

For some people, the experience of prejudice, harassment and persecution on the grounds of their sexuality means that making and sustaining personal relationships can be difficult. As well as general lesbian, gay and bisexual groups, there are specific groups for different communities including black and minority ethnic and religious groupings. The Lesbian and Gay Switchboard is one place where information about these groups can be found.

Participation

To vote or be a candidate in local government, regional and European elections in the UK, you need to be ordinarily resident or a UK or EU citizen, but for Westminster elections you need to be a British citizen or a citizen of another Commonwealth country or the Irish Republic (Eire).

As well as the formal electoral system, there are other opportunities to take part in civic life such as being a school or college governor, tenants or residents representative, magistrate or non-executive member of a health body (unless you work for the NHS) or joining the management committee of a voluntary organisation (including housing associations). Magistrates have to be citizens of the UK, Irish Republic or a Commonwealth country. Many of these (unpaid or token payment) appointments are advertised in local newspapers or *The Guardian* on Wednesdays. Appointments to other public (statutory) bodies are also advertised in newspapers but it helps to have registered an interest with the Public Appointments Commission. Public appointments are generally advertised at www.publicappts-vacs.gov.uk.

Resources

- The best place to find out about all the government agencies is on the Internet at www. open.gov.uk/Home/Homepage/fs/en. Many of the specific agencies mentioned in this chapter will be listed in their alphabetical index.

- To find out about how services in your area are organised, go to the website of your local authority. This is usually of the form www.localauthorityname.gov.uk

- To find out about voluntary organisations in your area go to www.nacvs.org.uk/cvsdir and look on the map for your area. Many refugee organisations are not formally linked to this network but the local umbrella group should be able to point you in the right direction www.ncvo-vol.org.uk

- For national (and some local) voluntary organisations go to www.ncvo-vol.org.uk and look in *About NCVO* for members.

- To find local Race Equality Council go to www.cre.gov.uk/about/recs.html

- For national refugee organisations go to www.refugeecouncil.org.uk or www.refugee-action.org

- For refugee organisations in your area go to the Refugee Community Organisation Development Project page at www.praxis.org.uk

- For organisations concerned with women's equality go to www.eoc.org.uk/EOCeng/dynpages/UsefulLinks.asp

- For Lesbian and Gay switchboards go to www.switchboard.org.uk

CHAPTER 6

IELTS provision

Tony Fitzgerald and Sam McCarter

What is IELTS?

The academic version of the International English Language Testing System or IELTS is the first step for doctors taking the Professional and Linguistic Assessment Board (PLAB) exam and those exempt from the PLAB. Candidates are examined in four skills: listening, writing, reading and speaking. Band scores ranging from 1 to 9 are given for each skill and a global mark is also given. Doctors taking the PLAB require a minimum global mark of 7. To achieve this they need at least three 7s and a 6, of which one 7 needs to be in speaking.

Listening module

The listening component of the IELTS comprises four extracts of spoken English, often dialogues or mini-lectures, for example an introductory lecture welcoming students onto a course or two students discussing timetables. The candidate is required to answer 10 questions (multiple choice, summary 'gap-fills', short answer questions or completing flow charts) on each extract. The extracts become more difficult as the test progresses.

The skills required here are:

- to read and understand the questions quickly prior to listening
- to listen and simultaneously record the key points heard
- to note correctly important numbers or dates mentioned
- to recognise subtle shades of expression
- to follow descriptions of procedures or processes.

Tips

- *Immerse yourself in spoken English as much as you can.* Listen regularly to radio and TV. Radio 4, for example, offers a range of broadcasts on current affairs, science, education and medicine in which you will encounter the type of vocabulary required in the test. Check your understanding of the news against the front-page stories in the broadsheets on the following day.

- *Make use of the vast amount of listening material that is available for students studying English at all levels.* For example, Cambridge Skills for Fluency 'Listening' Series, the 'Headway' or 'Cutting Edge' series ranging from elementary to advanced levels. These texts include listening materials and exercises very similar to those in the IELTS. Read the tasks, listen once and record your answers, check answers against the tapescripts/answer key.
- *Listen to material that includes people speaking in a variety of accents and styles.* The textbooks mentioned above include material of speakers using a range of accents, and speaking quickly, deliberately, with hesitations, etc.
- *Familiarise yourself with the way words are shortened, stressed and flow into each other in typical everyday speech.* 'Headway' has a series of books on pronunciation. It is important to be able to recognise how speakers may use stress and intonation patterns to indicate their attitude to what they are saying. Can you identify whether someone is speaking ironically, flippantly, with suppressed anger, etc.?

Academic reading module

This module lasts for 60 minutes and contains three reading passages, which may include pictures, graphs, tables or diagrams. The passages, which come from magazines, journals, books and newspapers, vary in length from approximately 500 to 1000 words with the total for the three being between 1500 and 2750. The reading texts cover general subjects, which do not require any specialist knowledge. Accompanying the passages, there are 40 questions. The texts and the questions become more difficult as you read from passage 1 to 3.

In this module, your reading comprehension skills are being tested, not your knowledge of any particular subject. The topics vary and are all of an academic nature. It is important to remember that the answers to all the questions are in the text itself. You do not need any knowledge of the topic to be able to answer the questions.

A limited range of questions is used to assess your understanding of the passages. The types of questions that normally occur are as follows.

Multiple choice questions

In MCQs, you are asked to choose the correct answer from four alternatives: ABCD. There are different ways to approach MCQs.

- Read the stem before you read the alternatives and give your own answer. As you read the alternatives, look for one to match your own answer.

- Find the alternatives which are not possible, because they are false or because no information is given about them.
- Cover the alternatives so that you can see only the stem. Then, reveal the alternatives one by one. In this way, you will become less confused.

Matching paragraph headings/sentences

In this type of exercise, you are asked to match a heading or a sentence with a paragraph. Many students find this type of question difficult. The following techniques may help you.

- Avoid reading just the first and last sentence of a paragraph to give you the heading. This does not work in many cases. It depends on the paragraph type.
- Read each paragraph quickly and then decide your own title. Then look for a heading with the same meaning in the exercise. If you read and decide at the same time, it only confuses you.
- Read a paragraph and ask yourself why it was written.
- Ask yourself if you can put all the information in the paragraph under the heading you have chosen.
- Check whether the heading contains words which are just lifted from the text. This may just be a distractor.
- Learn to distinguish between the *focus* of the paragraph and the *background information*, which is used to support the focus.
- Learn to recognise different types of paragraphs.
- Study the headings and try to predict what the paragraph for each heading is about. Or see if you can match all the headings with a theme, leaving out the distractors.
- Read the headings in the exercise first before you read the text.

Gap-filling exercises

There are basically two types of gap-filling exercise:

- a summary of the text or part of the text with a number of blank spaces, which you complete with a word or phrase from a word list
- a summary with a number of blank spaces without a word list, which you complete with words or phrases from the reading passage.

There are different techniques for doing this type of exercise. One is to read the summary through quickly to get the overall idea of the text. Then think of what kind of word you need for each blank space: an adjective, a noun, a verb, etc.

Think of your own words to complete the meaning of the text so that when you look at the reading passage or word list, you will recognise a synonym quicker.

Matching split sentences

Here candidates are asked to match the two parts of split sentences. Each completed sentence is usually a paraphrase of part of the text. So candidates have to look for synonyms in the reading passage. Make sure the grammar of the two parts fits.

The completion of sentences, summaries, diagrams, tables, flow charts, notes

This type of exercise usually tests candidates' ability to find and understand specific detail in a text. Candidates are asked to complete sentences or text by using a limited number of words taken from the passage. Note the text in the exercise is usually a paraphrase of the language in the reading passage. So you should not always be looking in the passage for the same words in the stem of the sentence, but the idea expressed in another way.

Short answers to open questions

This type of exercise is very similar to the previous one. Candidates need to check what the word limit is: it may be one, two, three or four words. Remember also to make sure that the words you choose fit the grammar of the sentences.

Yes/no/not given statements

This exercise asks you to analyse the passage by stating whether the information in a series of statements is correct, contradictory or if there is no information about the statement in the passage. Students find this type of question difficult. Read the whole statement carefully before you make a decision and make sure you look at the information in the whole statement, not part of it. Also make sure you use the question to analyse the text and not vice versa.

Hints on reading

Below are some hints about what you can do before the exam and during the exam.

- Spend only 20 minutes on each passage.
- Read the instructions carefully. It is important that candidates read all the instructions very carefully so that they are clear about what is required for the answer to each of the questions. A frequent mistake that candidates make is that they think that the instructions will be exactly the same as the textbook or other material they have been using for the exam.
- Read as widely as you can, newspapers, journals, specialist magazines and so on.
- Look for patterns in the organisation of texts. The different types of paragraphs are finite, but their arrangement can make them appear infinite in number.
- Read to understand the meaning of a passage rather than just the words.
- Learn to concentrate on the meaning, not the words, as you read.
- Always practise predicting what you are about to read.
- Try to summarise any text. This will then come to you automatically with practice.
- Increase your speed while still reading the organisation and meaning of a passage.
- Learn not to focus on words you do not know.
- Develop a series of strategies for marking texts as you read them.
- Remember that you have to transfer your answers from the question paper to your answer sheet within the 60 minutes.
- Spend a specific period each day reading.

Writing module

The academic module of the IELTS has two writing tasks. Task 1 requires the candidate to write a 'report' based on information presented in a diagram or chart. For instance, a graph might show the fluctuations in spending on different types of electronic equipment according to income group over a certain period. Alternatively, a flow chart could show the main stages in the design, production and marketing of a new type of television. The candidate is expected to write approximately 150 words in 20 minutes using the information presented as stimulus.

Task 2 asks the candidate to write an essay on a given topic of general interest. Topics that occur with some frequency include the effect of economic development on the environment, the importance of various aspects of education in society, the consequences of population growth and the impact of new technologies on individuals and societies.

In order to achieve a mark of at least 6 in the writing component, candidates must be able to write with a high degree of grammatical accuracy (which means that mistakes, where they occur, should not interfere with understanding), display a wide range of vocabulary and grammatical structures and be able to present a well-organised and logical argument.

For refugee doctors the writing component of the IELTS presents a number of challenges, but there is also much to gain from the learning/preparation for these tasks. We will consider first some of the particular challenges (i.e. what test candidates should and should not do) and then consider how this aspect of the test may benefit refugee doctors in terms of their general command of English as well as the particular skills they will require when they come to work in the UK.

Challenges

Different cultures and education systems place different degrees of importance and value on different types and styles of writing. In the UK, learning to write essays on general and academic topics has been a central aspect of education at secondary and tertiary level for many years. Essay writing is often a vital part of assessment and examination, especially in the subjects broadly defined as the 'humanities', such as history, literature and philosophy, and in the 'social sciences'. IELTS writing tasks, especially Task 2, grew out of this tradition and tend to be slanted towards topics and models of writing favoured in these two broad academic areas.

When tackling either of the writing tasks, keep in mind that *clarity of expression* is considered the essence of good writing. It is often said that the mark of a good writer is that s/he can convey even difficult ideas in a way that is readily comprehensible. This need for clarity applies at all levels of writing, affecting paragraph organisation, sentence structure and choice of vocabulary. How can this clarity be achieved?

General 'dos and don'ts': some tips that may help you with both tasks

- *Plan what you are going to write before you start to write.* It is essential that you draft an overall plan, indicating the topic of each paragraph and any examples you might use, before you commit pen to paper. All too often, nervous candidates begin to write before they have fully worked out what they are going to say. As a result, their 'reports' and essays may appear confused and lack logical development.

- *Try to ensure that each paragraph focuses on a single topic or theme.* Readers expect a paragraph to focus on one main idea, explaining the relevance of that idea and providing examples to support the point being made when appropriate. Readers will be confused by paragraphs where there is an abrupt shift between different ideas or topics.
- *Indicate the logical relationships within sentences.* In order to convey the logical relationships within sentences, you need to understand the use of 'conjunctions', i.e. words that link separate clauses so as to create a single sentence. Examples of conjunctions in English include 'and', 'but', 'so', 'if' and 'although'. You need to understand both the meaning of these words and the grammar and punctuation rules that apply when they are used.
- *Indicate the logical relationships between sentences.* In order to convey the logical relationships between sentences, you need to understand the use of 'connectors', i.e. words that indicate the relationship between the previous sentence(s) and the sentence(s) to follow. There are many more connectors in English than conjunctions. For example, there are connectors expressing sequence: 'first', 'then', 'next', 'finally'. Connectors that can express a cause/effect relationship: 'therefore', 'thus', 'consequently'. Or connectors of contrast: 'however', 'by contrast'. Once again, it is important that you understand the meaning of these words and the grammar and punctuation rules associated with their use.
- *Avoid 'run on'/long sentences.* Long sentences are more likely to be grammatically complex and difficult to control than short, pithy sentences. As a rule of thumb, one might say that sentences that contain more than one conjunction tend to be too long. A 'run on' sentence in English is one in which commas are used where full stops or a conjunction are required. This leads to the next 'do'.
- *Learn the rules of punctuation.* Rules of punctuation differ from one language to another, so it is essential that you understand when the common punctuation marks (full stops, commas, question marks, semi-colons and colons) can and cannot be used in English. Misuse of commas, in particular, is a frequent cause of lack of clarity when writing in English.
- *Avoid jargon or words that are unnecessarily obscure.* This may often be a matter of context or audience. What may seem to be medical jargon to a lay patient might be considered precise use of language by another doctor! Nevertheless, avoid using 'difficult' words simply to impress!
- *Don't allow the 'number of words requirement' to dictate the way you write.* Some candidates are so concerned about meeting the word targets (Task 1: 150; Task 2: 250) that they 'pad' sentences with unnecessary words that add nothing to the meaning. This frequently leads to grammar errors and a lack of clarity. Similarly, avoid phrasal verbs in favour of their single word synonym (e.g. 'let on' = 'inform/reveal') when possible.

Task 1: specific tips

- *Begin your report with a 'generalisation' based on the data presented in the chart.* Task 1 often presents candidates with data in the form of a chart/graph. Before starting to write, study the chart and decide on a single sentence that provides an overall analysis in general terms of the information contained in the chart. For example, with a chart that shows the sales of various types of electronic equipment over a 10-year period, you might begin:

  'It is clear that sales of video players and camcorders rose faster than sales of other types of electronic equipment from 1990 to 2000.'

  The generalisation presents an interpretation of the data in the chart. The remainder of your answer should select data from the chart that demonstrate the validity of your generalisation. You should not mention specific data in the generalisation.
- *Be clear about the tense or tenses required in your report.* For instance, if the chart shows data from a time that is finished, use simple past tense.
- *Bear in mind the form in which the data are presented.* Is the chart showing number or percentage? This may determine the grammatical structures you need to use. For example, if numbers are used, sentences beginning 'There are/were . . .' will probably be required.
- *Make sure you understand the grammar and meaning of the 'trend' verbs and adverbs.* The verbs include 'increase/decrease', 'rise/fall', 'raise/reduce'. Examples of relevant adverbs are 'slightly', 'gradually', 'significantly', 'markedly'.

Task 2: specific tips

- *Analyse the essay title before you start writing.* Is the title asking you to present your opinion on an issue? Does it require that you present reasons for and against a point of view? Is it asking that you consider the advantages and disadvantages of something? The answer to these questions should inform the way you structure your essay.
- *Decide on your opinion before you start to write.* If the essay title requires an opinion, don't decide on your view when you are writing your conclusion! It is essential that the reasons presented in the body of the essay provide support for your opinion. For this reason, it often helps to state your view clearly in the introduction to the essay.
- *Avoid exaggeration.* The following sentence presents an idea in an exaggerated way.

  'The use of computers leads to a reduction in face-to-face communication in all offices.'

It is not necessarily true that this is always the case! Two small changes in the sentence put the idea in proper perspective, i.e.

'The use of computers may lead to a reduction in face-to-face communication in many offices.'

- *Provide appropriate examples to support your view.* Try to provide examples that reinforce the points being made, and explain the relevance of the example.

Speaking module

The speaking section of the IELTS lasts between 11 and 14 minutes. During the examination you will have a conversation with an examiner, which is recorded. There are now three main parts within the oral exam.

1 *Introduction.* You and the examiner introduce yourselves to one another. The examiner will try to put you at your ease and check your identity and ask you questions which are taken from one of a number of topic frames: your studies, your family life, etc. This section lasts 4–5 minutes.
2 *Individual long turn.* You will speak to the examiner about a particular topic for 1–2 minutes. This will include an explanation, description or narration. For example, you may be asked to describe the person who has influenced you most in your life. The topic is written on a card with a few prompts. You are given one minute to prepare before you speak at length for 1–2 minutes. Afterwards the examiner will ask you a few questions. This section lasts 3–4 minutes.
3 *Two-way discussion.* You will have a discussion with the examiner about a topic linked to Part 2. The questions asked will be of a more abstract nature. The length of the discussion is 4–5 minutes.

General points about the speaking module

- In the speaking module, the examiner is assessing whether you can *communicate effectively in English.* The examiner is therefore testing not just your grammatical accuracy but also the communicative strategies you use and whether your grammar and vocabulary are appropriate and flexible.
- Students often make the mistake of learning chunks of information by heart. This causes problems, because it is very easy for an examiner to see if you are doing this. The examiner can check your fluency by asking a question you are not prepared for!
- You need to give the examiner enough evidence of your ability to use English in communication. Otherwise, you will probably not receive the score you deserve. You should, therefore, learn to develop your answers to the examiner's questions.

Where IELTS fits in

Many doctors see the IELTS as a hurdle, but many also say that they realise its value when they come to take Part 2 of the PLAB exam. Parts 1 and 2 of the PLAB test a candidate's experience as a doctor. The IELTS tests candidates' skill and competence in English, not their knowledge of the language. The IELTS therefore fits in to the same pathway.

CHAPTER 7

Learning needs assessment

Anwar Khan and Jeanette Naish

Introduction

Arriving in a new country as a refugee must be a difficult time. There will be bewildering regulations about where and how to live. Families are uprooted and familiar social and community networks no longer exist. A new life has to be built, as well as a new career.

To address the career, the first thing that needs understanding is what the 'licensing' authority requires. In the United Kingdom, that authority is the General Medical Council. It would serve the aspiring refugee doctor wishing to practise in the UK healthcare system to find out the necessary information and to understand that information, in order to plan the process that will inevitably be required to achieve that aspiration.

In a strange country, with a strange healthcare system, unfamiliar medical culture and public expectations, there will be many new things that have to be learned in terms of knowledge, skills and attitudes. Like all learners in the medical fraternity, refugee doctors will be at different stages of learning. They will therefore have particular learning needs. These may well be different from those of doctors educated in the UK. It is therefore essential that refugee doctors identify what it is that they need to learn and what is relevant to their future careers. Educators equally need to understand what these learning needs are, so that syllabus and learning opportunities are formulated to meet them.

Purpose of learning needs assessment

From the learner's point of view, a learning needs assessment is an attempt to identify the gap between existing knowledge, skills and attitudes and those that are needed in order to carry out their daily work appropriately. Assessing learning needs has a fundamental role in education and training to ensure the relevance of the educational activity to the learners.[1,2] If educators disregard the needs of learners, they may not know what the learners need to learn, what is relevant and what will motivate them to learn.

Identifying need

By whom and how learning needs are assessed will depend on the purpose of the assessment. The needs of adult learners engaged in postgraduate professional education can be classified by two main criteria: who is determining the needs (learners, educators or others) and what standards are used as the ideal.

For the refugee doctor, the assessment will be driven by the requirement of their 'high-stakes' examinations, namely the IELTS and PLAB. For the educator, learning needs assessment might be used to help to plan the curriculum, help the individual plan their education, assess learning, or demonstrate improved practice. Published classifications[1-4] of 'needs' include the following.

- Within a group of learners, *felt needs* (or *perceived needs*) are what the individual or the group have identified as what they want to learn. Their knowledge, experience and the environment they work in influence most of these needs. These are the learner's needs as *perceived* by the learner and are characterised by the sentence, 'I know what I don't know'.
- *Expressed needs* are what an individual or group express as their needs. Not all perceived needs are expressed because there may be several real or perceived barriers to expression. For example, learners may not want to be identified as lacking knowledge or they may lack the opportunity to express their needs. Learners may also lack the motivation, communication skills or assertiveness to express their needs. This lack of expression (or demand) can create an unhealthy situation, because it can be confused with the absence of a need for a particular educational intervention.
- *Normative needs* are defined as the measured gap between the set standards and the individual's or group's current knowledge. The standards are set by experts in a particular field, for example expert committees of the General Medical Council or the Royal Colleges.* The opinion of those being assessed is not taken into account.
- *Comparative needs* are those learning needs identified by comparing two similar groups or individuals rather than against normative standards.

---

* In the United Kingdom, the Royal Colleges are academic and administrative bodies representing the different medical specialties; for example, the Royal College of Physicians, Royal College of General Practitioners, Royal College of Surgeons and so on. Their principal role is to set standards for practice so that they convene structured assessments: examinations for registered practitioners in each specialty, for entry into the Royal Colleges. On the other hand, the General Medical Council is the body responsible for regulation of practice and for issuing the licence to practise.

- *Prescribed needs* are identified by educators or programme planners for individuals (or groups) who fail to meet a predetermined standard of performance. The reason for this failure is generally attributed to gaps in the knowledge, skills or attitudes needed for high-quality performance. An educational programme for remediation is then 'prescribed' to address this gap. They usually take normative needs into account.
- *Unperceived needs* are gaps in learning that the learner is not aware of and may be characterised by the sentence, 'I don't know what I don't know' (Johari's window – see below).

Methods for learning needs assessment

Learning needs may be clinical versus administrative needs or even subjective versus objectively measured needs. The defined purpose of the needs assessment should determine the method used and how to use findings. Gaps in learning can be identified using objective or subjective tools and each of the tools has its strengths and weaknesses. Objective tools tend to assess knowledge rather than skills and attitudes. Multiple choice examinations are a typical example of objective assessment of knowledge. Other methods include questionnaires, confidence rating scales and so on (see below).

It would be unrealistic to expect that assessing learning needs can be done as one overarching exercise. Different ways of doing this are required for different domains of learning.

Needs of the learner

On arrival in the UK

Refugee doctors have arrived in the UK not through choice but of necessity. Consequently, their learning could be hampered by other more pressing issues such as settling in a new country.

Levels of learning need

Maslow[5] postulated the hierarchy of needs (Figure 7.1), suggesting that human beings are motivated by unsatisfied needs and certain basic levels of need have to be satisfied before higher needs can be dealt with. As the person progresses from the lower to higher levels, learning takes place, leading to intellectual growth and development. Maslow believed that people should be able to move through the needs to the highest level provided that they are given an education that promotes growth.

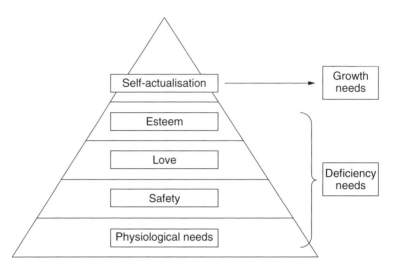

Figure 7.1   Maslow's hierarchy of needs.

With regard to refugee doctors, their 'physiological' needs include basic ones such as food and shelter; the housing and financial difficulties they face are significant and often cause delay in their return to work in medicine.

The 'safety' needs relate to establishing stability and consistency in a chaotic world. Not only is there legal wrangling over their immigration status, which adds to the uncertainty of the situation, but the angst is compounded by worry about families elsewhere whose fate may be uncertain.

The 'love' needs revolve around a desire to belong to groups and be accepted by others.

'Esteem' needs are to do with self-esteem that is gained by competence and mastery of tasks and the esteem gained from the attention and recognition coming from others.

Maslow felt that the basic 'deficiency' needs have to be met before the person can progress onto 'growth' needs, when the individual has a 'desire to become more and more what one is, to become everything that one is capable of becoming'. Self-actualisation is characterised by:

- being problem focused
- incorporating ongoing freshness of experience of life
- having a concern regarding personal growth
- ability to reach one's peak potential.

Some of the changes in the educational process that Maslow espoused included:

- people should transcend their cultural conditioning
- they should learn from their inner nature.

Language issues

A significant hurdle is the IELTS examination, the content of which is far removed from refugee doctors' aspirations of continuing their career in medicine. It seems that a significant number choose to pursue other career choices since they cannot make the required grade in the IELTS examination. Many find that the IELTS tests esoteric subject matter and this lack of relevance affects their ability to learn. The purpose of the language course is to 'master' the English language for IELTS but the refugee doctors need to learn 'medical' English. The best way to learn to read is to read, regardless of what the set reading is. The best way to learn a spoken language is to hear it and speak it, but there are very few opportunities for these doctors to do this, particularly in the medical context. Placing this language training in the context of clinical attachments allows some relevance to be seen by the learners.

Past learning experiences

With regard to refugee doctors' past learning experiences, their training is often in a system very different to the one they encounter in this country and the skills gained previously may not be relevant in the modern NHS.

Experience of patient management

In their own countries, they will have encountered differing morbidities and hence have differing priorities when dealing with patients. There is more chronic disease in the UK while infectious diseases are more prevalent in their countries of origin. The doctor–patient interaction is more of a curative role rather than the greater duty of care that chronic disease management entails. One doctor commented, 'The relationship is more of a friend' with a greater emphasis on social aspects than just dealing with the medical aspects of the case. There is a greater degree of patient involvement in management in the UK as compared to their past experiences. In their countries, being 'doctor centred' shows more authority and knowledge whilst 'patient-centred' consulting demonstrates a lack of knowledge on the doctor's part; the patient has come for a medical opinion and should be 'told what to do'.

There are also differences in technology. The more sophisticated and advanced technology will be unknown to some refugee doctors. Not just what the tests/treatments are but the physiological basis for them. The refugee doctors will inevitably have gaps in their knowledge and skills (including health promotion/health education/communication skills).

Learning style

Refugee doctors are no different from other adult learners who exhibit the following main characteristics.[6]

- They have a purpose for their education and have expectations about the learning process.
- They are not beginners and they bring their own unique experiences and values.
- They have developed their own set patterns of learning.
- They have competing interests such as bringing up a family, etc.

Knowles[7] believed that adult learners needed to feel a necessity to learn and that identifying one's own learning needs was an essential part of self-directed learning. What motivates a person to learn? A number of factors (such as personality, learning styles, etc.) interact but essentially, we must engage them in the learning process, using their past experiences, and the learning activities need to be relevant to their circumstances. Hence, it is essential that we have a holistic approach and account for their differing motivation, circumstances, individual learning needs and learning styles.

Approaches to teaching

As educators, we need to be aware that different people learn in different ways and this leads to the concept of learning styles; five different models are summarised in *Educating the Future GP* by McEvoy.[8] In one model, Honey and Mumford[9] described four different learning types.

- *Activist* – these people are open-minded and often welcome new ideas and experiences but are bored with implementation and longer term consolidation.
- *Reflector* – they are cautious people who consider implications, gather the data and think about it thoroughly before coming to any conclusion.
- *Theorist* – these integrate new material into logical sound theories. They tend to be perfectionists who incorporate learning with their experiences. They are uncomfortable with subjective arguments and prefer certainty.
- *Pragmatist* – these types try out new knowledge to see if it works in practice.

We are not exclusively one or other of the groups but have a mixture of learning styles. It is important to know what works for each individual and both learners and educators would benefit from getting an idea of their learning style since this has an effect on the teaching style.

Learners may be used to a teacher–pupil hierarchy system with a structured and didactic approach to learning. Questioning the 'teacher' may be difficult for some of them to get used to. Consequently, they may be unfamiliar with teaching methods employed in the UK with respect to 'learning sets' and 'self-directed' learning and problem-based learning may be more appropriate.

Educating the reflective doctor

In the UK, we value the reflective learner but overseas doctors feel uncomfortable with reflection. But this can and should be learned. The domains of the mind are only expressed if stimulated, either through training, as in pedagogic learning, or through vocational requirements. For example, highly convergent, rapid problem-solving domains are expressed because of vocational needs in GPs. On the other hand, abstract thinking in academics involves divergent thinking about the many aspects of a single problem. Reflective thinking is suppressed until later in life when these domains are allowed to develop. Kolb's model of the learning cycle[10] refers to the process by which individuals attend to and understand their experiences and consequently modify their behaviours. It is based on the idea that the more often we reflect on a task, the more often we have the opportunity to modify and refine our efforts. The learning cycle contains the following four stages.

- *Experiencing* or *immersing oneself in the 'doing'* of a task is the first stage in which the individual simply carries out the task assigned. The engaged person is usually not reflecting on the task at this time, but carrying it out with intention.
- *Reflection* involves stepping back from task involvement and *reviewing what has been done* and experienced. The skills of attending, noticing differences and applying terms help identify subtle events and communicate them clearly to others. One's paradigm (values, attitudes, beliefs) influences whether one can differentiate certain events. One's vocabulary is also influential since without words, it is difficult to verbalise and discuss one's perceptions.
- *Conceptualisation* involves *interpreting the events* that have been noticed and *understanding the relationships* among them. It is at this stage that theory may be particularly helpful as a template for framing and explaining events. One's paradigm again influences the interpretive range a person is willing to entertain.
- *Planning* includes taking the new understanding and translating it into *predictions* about what is likely to happen next or *what actions should be taken* to refine the way the task is handled.

Cultural differences

A common observation of refugee doctors is that in the UK, 'the family is not supportive' as compared to their experiences in their own countries. They find it difficult to understand how an elderly relative can be left in a home without any family involvement. They feel that they must not assume family support when dealing with patients. Maintaining confidentiality may be anathema to them when they have been used to extended families that share their experiences.

Teenage pregnancies are a case in point; discussion about a pregnant 15-year-old schoolgirl highlighted their surprise as to how she was made to feel relaxed by the doctor about her decision to have a termination in a non-judgemental manner, without the necessity of informing the parents. The management was about focusing on future care and emphasising it was 'not the end of the world'.

Learning in the UK

Refugee doctors come from a number of backgrounds but their medical knowledge is the common thread and they have similar learning needs when they come to the UK.

Confidence and competence

Confidence rating scales can be used to help doctors identify their needs. These are lists of topics that aim to cover the content of general practice, which is vast! The learners score themselves on the level of confidence reached in a particular subject. They are useful to identify potentially weak areas but do need honest self-assessment which can be difficult to do early in one's career. Later, the more we learn, the more we realise there is to learn and hence doctors may not fill this in consistently during the training period. The subject matter that has been pre-determined may not be up to date, especially if the scales were developed many years previously.

The use of competence rating scales again involves supplying a list of topics but this time the educator scores the learner. The original vocational training rating scale was developed by the University of Manchester in 1976 but was replaced by a modified and shortened questionnaire in 1989. Another tool is the Barnet Assessment Form which was developed in 1997. However, they are tedious to complete and are a subjective assessment by the educator. The results need to be used for information and development rather than judgement; a significant degree of tact and sensitivity is needed by the educator. Dr Tim Swanwick[11] provides a good introduction to the formative assessment toolbox.

Learning from patients

There does seem to be a need to provide more training in a clinical attachment setting to allow doctors to become acquainted with the NHS and also to provide a link to their studies, in particular for the PLAB examinations.

In relation to learning with respect to patient care, the areas in medicine that have been highlighted as needing particular attention include the following.

- *Care of the elderly.* This is the most requested specialty since very few have experience of it; not many people in their countries have reached such an age.

- *Psychiatry.* Transcultural factors play a significant part as well as understanding of language. There is the theory that illness is socially constructed; therefore it is hardly surprising that refugee doctors from some cultures do not recognise mental illness, let alone understand the Western perception of mental ill health.
- *Paediatrics.* More chronic conditions in the UK.
- *Obstetrics and gynaecology.* Some, particularly male, doctors have very little experience of this specialty.
- *Ethics.* See above under cultural aspects.
- *Guidelines and protocols.* It was felt that this allowed setting of boundaries and highlighted major incentives to health (e.g. cholesterol screening) and hence increased quality of practice in the UK.
- *Doctor–patient relationship.* The overseas doctors need to adapt from a doctor-centred and paternalistic style, that they have been used to in the past, to a patient-centred approach involving negotiation with patients. In the UK, this is based on professionalism with humanity, confidentiality, listening and communication skills, dealing with uncertainty/anger/crisis/complaints and a holistic picture of the patient with multiple dimensions (family, occupation, hidden agendas and learned illness behaviour).

Self-knowledge: developing insights and awareness of gaps in learning

It is in the context of seeing patients that the doctors can be helped in identifying their learning needs. In order to do this, one requires some honest reflection, self-assessment on the part of the learner and use of structured methods by the educator.

The various states of self-knowledge are succinctly summarised by the Johari window (Fig. 7.2). The Johari window was named after the first names of its inventors, Joseph Luft and Harry Ingham, and is very useful in identifying learning needs.[12] A four-paned 'window' divides personal awareness into four different types, as represented by its four quadrants: open, hidden, blind and unknown. The lines dividing the four panes are like window shades, which can move as an interaction progresses. In this model, each person is represented by their own window.

	Known to self	Unknown to self
Known to others	*Open*	*Blind*
Unknown to others	*Hidden*	*Unknown*

Figure 7.2 The Johari window.

- The *open* quadrant represents things that both the learner and educator know about the learner. This can include not only factual information but also feelings, motives, behaviours, wants, needs, etc. The process of enlarging the open quadrant is called self-disclosure.
- The *blind* quadrant represents things that the educator knows but the learner does not.
- The *hidden* quadrant represents things that the learner knows but the educator does not.
- The *unknown* quadrant represents things that neither the learner nor educator knows about the learner.

The process of moving previously unknown information into the open quadrant, thus enlarging its area, has been likened to Maslow's concept of self-actualisation.

Understanding and accepting the need to learn

The aim of identifying learning needs is to expand the 'open' box quadrant so that the learner knows what he or she does not know and the educator can be aware of those deficiencies. For this to occur there needs to be a relationship based on trust and openness so that disclosure is both possible and safe and things in the 'hidden' quadrant (i.e. inadequacies known only to the learner) can be brought out into the daylight and dealt with effectively. As one's level of confidence and self-esteem develops, one may actively invite others to comment on one's blind spots. The use of more structured formative assessment tools allow us to gain an insight into 'blind' and 'unknown' quadrants. In identifying learning needs, we do need to balance the learner's learning 'wants' and learning 'needs'.

PUNS and DENS is a method of highlighting educational needs in the surgery setting and was developed by Dr Richard Eve in 1995.[13] It is all too tempting to just learn more about the things we are interested in and probably have a good knowledge base about already. Dr Eve's idea was that for learning to be relevant and improve our service, it should be patient driven. It addresses the patient's needs that are not being met (Patient Unmet Needs) as a direct result of the doctor's lack of knowledge or skill (Doctor's Educational Needs).

Recording patient contact

The PUNS and DENS method involves keeping a logbook of patient consultations which should highlight a number of areas of need. Having identified and written down the PUNs, the learner considers *why* the patient's needs went unmet, annotates the deficiencies identified in him/herself and writes down an action plan to remedy the situation. It does not aim to address 'wants' from the patient or learner but rather 'needs'. It is possible not only to identify gaps in knowledge by this method but also to understand why an individual finds certain patients difficult and hence help people understand how they can become more effective in their work. However, the process of logging or recording can be subjective.

Sharing learning

Sharing the experience of managing cases with peers is an important and valuable opportunity for learning. Case discussions are indispensable since each patient is a potential learning experience; they are rooted in real life and the personal experience of the learners. In problem case analysis, the learner brings records of patients who are interesting or causing difficulties whilst in random case analysis, the learner brings the notes of a complete surgery and cases are picked at random. The resulting discussions highlight the real questions and how to deal with them. The discussion around practical solutions can end up covering areas of need far distant from the original perceived problem. It does need some honest reflections on the part of the learner. As well as hitherto undiscovered learning needs being revealed, it can provide the motivation to enhance the learning experience.

Learning from mistakes

Significant event analysis (SEA) is a method of learning from our mistakes and thereby highlighting those learning needs in the 'hidden' quadrant of the Johari window. A significant event such as a missed diagnosis, death of a patient or a practice complaint is brought to the attention of the learner. All the parties involved discuss why the event is considered significant and determine the facts of the case in order to tease out the important issues raised by the event. What went well is highlighted together with what went badly and areas for improvement are identified so as to draw up an action plan. For this method to succeed it should be a positive experience for all involved in spite of highlighting areas that need improvement. The overriding ethos should be that it is about improvement and development rather than blame.

The patient's viewpoint

Patients are a valuable source of feedback and we could use a patient satisfaction questionnaire. However, there is a tendency for patients to comment on the 'niceness' of a doctor rather than competence. Formal instruments such as the Howie Enablement Questionnaire might be useful in this respect.

The Follow-Up Slip System (FUSS) is a simple means of rapidly collecting information on learners' performance. In this method, FUSS cards are lodged in the notes of a number of consecutive patients and these are pulled out and completed by the next doctor seeing that patient. That doctor then comments on the diagnosis, management and patient's impression of the previous consultation. These cards are returned and can be analysed for trends, e.g. recurring mistakes in a particular area. Some adaptation will be needed for paperless practices. The educator then provides feedback to the learner.

The consultation

Mutual exploration of the issues generated by videoed consultation is one of the most powerful formative tools available in GP training. The value of the use of video cannot be overemphasised; after all, the consultation is the cornerstone of general practice and all else follows from it.

In recent years there has been a growth industry in consultation rating scales. One can assess consultations by looking at the *outcomes* of the various phases, e.g. was a rapport established? Was the problem identified? Was time used well? Alternatively one can assess the *process* and the *behaviour* of the doctor, e.g. how was the patient greeted? How was information elicited (were open or closed questions used)? How much was the consultation oriented towards the patient rather than the doctor?

Assessing performance during consultations

Peter Tate has suggested a series of questions to ask yourself after the consultation (details on the RCGP website: www.rcgp.org.uk), which are as follows.

- Do I know significantly more about them than before they came in the door?
- Was I curious?
- Did I listen?
- Did I explore their agenda, beliefs and expectations?
- Did I make an acceptable working diagnosis?
- Did I use what they thought when I started explaining?
- Did I share options for investigations or treatments?
- Did I involve them in decision making?
- Did I make some attempt to ensure that they really understood?
- Was I friendly?

There are a number of consultation analysis tools available and a valuable introduction is provided by Peter Tate's book.[14]

Peer observation

Joint surgeries are an excellent source of learning needs but having another person in the consultation can affect both the process and outcome of that consultation. Patients also find it hard to ignore the fact that a more experienced and more familiar doctor is in the room and may begin to address their enquiries in that direction. Using these joint surgeries for both the trainer and learner to bring back 'problem cases' adds to the ethos of joint learning. Watching a learner consult with the use of a 'live-link' gets round the problem of too many in the consultation room, but there are ethical considerations around both the learner and patient alike.

Audit is a powerful tool in that it is about what we actually do, not what we say we do or know. It compares our performance against a set of criteria and standards. Encouraging the learner to conduct small-scale focused audits on a regular basis is a very good way of identifying failings and improving the quality of care delivered.

Feedback

Remember that the purpose of feedback is to help the learner to become aware of how s/he performs a particular task. It should not be seen as an opportunity to criticise the person. Feedback can be given, and accepted, well or badly and it is useful to have rules for sensitive feedback. Pendleton's rules or a variation are usually employed, but the important thing is to comment on fact and to point out things that can be changed. It is helpful to suggest an alternative action rather than just pointing out what you think is wrong.

- The doctor whose work is being considered usually says what s/he thinks s/he did well.
- The colleague then points out what was well done and perhaps why.
- In this phase of the feedback it is usually difficult to get the right balance as these doctors have been used to destructive criticism and opinions from their 'teachers'. They have commented that, in the UK, sometimes they feel feedback can be 'too sensitive and dovish'.
- The doctor whose work is being considered then says what s/he might have done differently or better and why.
- Next the colleague helps with sensitively voiced suggestions about what can be done differently.
- Finally it is useful for the doctor whose work is being considered to think about the meeting a few days later and maybe try out one of the suggestions.

Ideally, the educator will give positive feedback where it is due and strive to achieve mutual agreement with the learner when offering constructive criticism. When things aren't going so well, it is helpful for the educator to know if there are any external factors, e.g. difficulty with a colleague might be affecting performance at work.

Assessment-driven learning

As with other groups studying for examinations, the syllabus of the examination in question (e.g. PLAB and IELTS) will drive their learning and hence pose barriers to real learning. In view of the language difficulties, there are particular learning needs in preparation for the examinations; for example, the MCQ component is highlighted as a major problem.

Multiple choice questions

Multiple choice questions are probably the best method of testing knowledge. They have the advantages of high reliability and rapidity of scoring with economy of staff time as well as being able to sample large content areas. The move away from simple true–false statements to more complex question formats, such as extended matching questions and single and multiple best answer questions, will allow testing of the understanding and application of knowledge rather than just factual acquisition itself. The PEP (Phased Evaluation Project) is a computerised MCQ (available from the RCGP) which tests factual knowledge in a number of areas. The participant's scores are compared with pooled results. However, the questions set need to be validated and also only test competence rather than performance.

Objective structured clinical examination

Objective structured clinical examinations (OSCEs) are being used increasingly as endpoint assessments at medical school, summative assessment and PLAB examinations. The candidate is consulted by a simulated patient who has carefully rehearsed common scenarios compatible with the learner's expected areas of knowledge, skill and practice. A marking schedule is prepared in advance for scoring the way each consultation is handled. However, OSCEs need lots of preparation and detailed briefing of role players. We have found that the use of simulated patients is fun and well received by the refugee doctors. They have found it to be educational in being able to try out different consultation techniques and get feedback from the simulated patient, which is then incorporated into the learning experience.

Future planning

Passing the PLAB is 'not the end of the story' since it is the beginning of the search for appropriate jobs. In their own countries, refugee doctors are allocated jobs rather than going through an application process, which is common in the UK. Consequently, they have not been used to applying for jobs. There is a particular need to get used to 'job-hunting' in the UK, which in turn requires skills in CV writing and interview techniques. Having a mentor to provide timely career advice is a luxury that few have access to and hence they may be dejected by lack of success in their numerous applications for jobs. Organisations such as RETAS can help in this regard.

An appraisal is a formative assessment process that gives the learner an opportunity to reflect on the educational experience as well as providing a forum to review what has been accomplished and plan for future learning. Appraisals are about 'praise' and development and should end with a mutually agreed statement of where future energies should be directed and an action plan. Objectives should be SMART: specific, measurable, attainable, resourced and time bounded.

Conclusion

Refugee doctors need help to learn how to learn. This involves doing an adequate 'needs' assessment, beyond the needs of the PLAB examination, by inviting their curiosity to identify areas of learning. An appreciation of their motivation to learn, personality profiles, barriers in their personal lives and learning styles is essential. This will allow them to expand their repertoire of study skills and so help select the most effective approach to learning for the individual. Goal setting allows learners to become actively involved in the learning process and they are then able to clarify for themselves their strengths and weaknesses. The aim of autonomous and life-long learning can be aided by appropriate use of information technology. Problem-based learning has been shown to have lasting influence on learning behaviour. The educator/mentor can help in drawing conclusions for continuing learning as a form of portfolio. This portfolio-based learning has the advantage of being learner centred as well as encouraging deep learning.

The proper use of formative assessment methods should have the aim of promoting the autonomy of the learner, developing openness and encouraging life-long learning.

Acknowledgement

Our thanks to Dr Penny Trafford, whose advice and support have been invaluable.

References

1 Grant J (2002) Learning needs assessment: assessing the need. *BMJ.* **324**: 156–9.

2 Ratnapalan S and Hilliard RI (2002) Needs assessment in postgraduate medical education: a review. *Med Educ Online.* **7**: 8.

3 Davis DA (1998) Global health, global learning. *BMJ.* **316**: 385–9.

4 Myers P (1999) The objective assessment of general practitioners' educational needs: an under-researched area? *Br J Gen Pract.* **49**: 303–7.

5 Maslow AH (1998) *Toward a Psychology of Being* (3e). Wiley, New York.

6 Brookfield S (1985) The continuing educator and self-directed learning in the community. In: S Brookfield (ed.) *Self-Directed Learning: from theory to practice.* New Directions for Continuing Education No. 25. Jossey-Bass, San Francisdco.

7 Knowles N (1990) *The Adult Learner: a neglected species* (4e). Gulf, Houston.

8 McEvoy P (1998) *Educating the Future GP: the Course Organisers Handbook* (2e). Radcliffe Medical Press, Oxford.

9 Honey P and Mumford A (1982) *Manual of Learning Styles.* P Honey, London.

10 Kolb David A (1984) *Experimental Learning: experience as the source of learning and development.* Prentice-Hall Inc., Englewood Cliffs, NJ.

11 Swanwick T. Formative Assessment Toolbox. http://www.londondeanery.ac.uk/gp/home.htm

12 Luft J and Ingham H (1955) The Johari Window: a graphic model for interpersonal relations. University of California Western Training Lab.

13 Eve R (2000) Learnng with PUNs and DENs: a method for determining educational needs and the evaluation of its use in primary care. *Educ Gen Pract.* **11**: 73–9.

14 Tate P (2002) *The Doctors Communication Handbook* (4e). Radcliffe Medical Press, Oxford.

CHAPTER 8

Running PLAB study groups

*Jo Scrivens, Sheila Cheeroth and
Geoff Norris*

Introduction

Refugee doctors are often unable to continue their careers because they have difficulty in overcoming the financial, educational and professional barriers to practice. Refugee doctors have qualified overseas and may not practise in the UK before passing an English test (the International English Language Testing System or IELTS) followed by a medical examination (the Professional and Linguistic Assessment Board or PLAB test) as stipulated by the General Medical Council. The PLAB test checks that overseas doctors have the basic medical knowledge and skills to work at SHO level in the NHS. There are relatively few courses and most are prohibitively expensive to refugee doctors.

Study groups can be invaluable; refugee doctors can pool their information, expertise and resources to stimulate study and support each other, relieving what is sometimes crippling isolation. Support from the NHS or other agencies can make this process much easier and far more productive. Overseas qualified doctors with settled status often also face hardship in getting through similar barriers. Whether or not they are included in clubs depends on the motivation of the supporters (for example workforce development confederations often view this as a recruitment issue) and the pressure on the study club's resources. Where, as in London, the need for educational support from internationally qualified doctors outstrips supply, there is often a tendency to limit the study club membership in some way, sometimes by barring non-refugees. In other areas of the country, the non-refugee doctors sometimes contribute to the critical mass of members needed to make the meetings work well. Certainly it is interesting to note that the NHS is currently recruiting abroad for doctors, a not inexpensive venture.

Study clubs: aims, objectives and allied objectives

Study groups are groups of doctors who meet to study together, in this case primarily for the PLAB examination.

Some have been founded by request of refugee doctors with support of local doctors or agencies, some have been formed and are run almost entirely by migrant/refugee doctors. They can range from the entirely self-directed (often called discussion groups by the doctors in them) to those with a set repeating timetable that aims to cover the PLAB syllabus. Most often they are something in between, with a facilitator trying to both set the programme to respond to the expressed learning needs of the members and guide the club members to ensure that a good cross-section of the required material is covered. Usually if there is an NHS doctor as a facilitator, the time available for meeting is restricted to two hours weekly. In our experience meetings need to take place a minimum of fortnightly to maintain momentum.

Aims

- To assist refugee doctors to re-enter their profession in the UK by providing a forum for peer support. Refugee doctors can pool their information, expertise and resources to stimulate study and support each other, relieving what is sometimes crippling isolation and the sterility of studying for a medical examination with no contact with patients or the profession.
- To provide direct educational support to doctors in studying for the IELTS and PLAB examinations.

Objectives

- Provide opportunities to develop spoken and listening English language skills that can contribute to their performance in the IELTS.
- Provide opportunities to develop specifically medical English communication skills necessary for the PLAB. For this it is particularly useful to have access to a doctor practising in the NHS.
- Provide opportunities to update medical knowledge.
- Help members to become familiar with the UK medical environment, e.g. ethical issues, working practices, patterns of pathology in the local population.
- Provide opportunities to become familiar with the UK medical examination system by discussing examination questions.

- Act as a forum for discussion of opportunities for appropriate and accessible English language and medical education opportunities elsewhere.

Optional/peripheral aims and objectives

Liaison

Refugees are very much an excluded group and it is difficult for them to access facilities. The intervention of an NHS doctor can help enormously.

Organising access to literature

Refugee doctors cannot afford journals and medical textbooks and are not generally allowed to use hospital medical libraries. The facilitator can ask a public library if they will stock a small collection of books appropriate for the PLAB. The Westminster Public Library took advice on this from one of the authors (SC) a few years ago when it was decided it would be the one public library in London to stock medical textbooks often used for the PLAB.

In other cases facilitators have liaised with the local postgraduate medical centre to arrange access for their club members. The regional postgraduate deaneries all have a dean with responsibilities for overseas and refugee doctors and they may be able to exert influence here.

An obstetrics and gynaecology registrar, one of the regular contributors to teaching at the East London Study Club (run by SC), took it upon herself to persuade her hospital's pharmacy department to give the study club excess copies of the *British National Formulary*. Many BNFs are not used after one year when they would still be extremely useful for PLAB preparation.

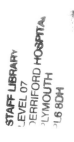

Organising access to existing continuing medical education meetings

Facilitators may be able to access local educational meetings for refugee doctors via the local GP tutor and the local hospital postgraduate tutor.

Developing links with other agencies

Other local agencies may be able to meet the needs of refugee doctors that the study club cannot help with. Agencies that may help include:

- the local adult education sector which might provide English language courses
- employment and training organisations, both voluntary and statutory, with advice on benefits, educational opportunities and English courses
- community organisations

- health authorities and primary care organisations
- postgraduate medical centres
- postgraduate deaneries which should have a dean with designated responsibility for education and training for overseas and refugee doctors.

In order to maximise the potential of any study club, it is necessary to be flexible in how they are run due to issues around resources (facilitator availability, accommodation) and specific characteristics particular to each individual group of doctors (size of group, stage in progress towards registration).

Even study groups that have no regular NHS doctor to facilitate meetings will benefit enormously from having a champion, whether a doctor or not. There is a great deal of scope for truly self-directed learning groups. Where these have been set up, they have flourished; for example, there is one that meets at St Thomas' Hospital in London for four hours six days a week. A similar group met at International Student House in Great Portland Street for many years, 2–3 times a week. These groups flourished simply on word of mouth and in fact, often they were victims of their own success, becoming too large to function easily and having to limit publicity to prevent overgrowth. The key factors for success seem to be the availability of a frequent consistent regular study space (a meeting room with a table and seating for 8–12 is usually sufficient) and good public transport links.

The rest of this chapter will focus on study clubs facilitated by a doctor practising in the NHS.

Formulating an educational framework/timetable

Before deciding on an educational framework or timetable it is important to consider the aims and objectives of the students attending the study group. The most important aim for most individuals will be to pass Parts 1 and 2 of the PLAB exam and, rightly or wrongly, other aims and objectives will be of less relevance until the exam is passed. The programme that will be most enthusiastically received will be one that concentrates on the most frequent topics appearing in the exam. As the GMC does not publish past papers, most of this information relies on past exam students recalling the questions they were asked. Other sources of information are included under Resources below. Since the PLAB exam aims to ensure that the overseas qualified doctor is able to successfully undertake an SHO post in the NHS hospital setting, the learning should be pitched at this level and oriented to the practical issues facing the SHO.

Another area worth considering for some time on the schedule is information and skilling up for job searching.

Teaching methods

Detailed information about different teaching techniques and methods can be obtained from relevant textbooks on these subjects. Below is a list of methods that have been fruitfully used in study clubs. The success of these will depend on the experience of the tutor/facilitator, the confidence of the refugee doctors within their study group setting, the size of the group and the willingness of the group to participate in teaching techniques that may be new to them.

- Didactic teaching by study group tutor or specialist outside speaker, e.g. 'Common ENT problems presenting to the SHO'.
- Video viewing to learn examination techniques followed by practice in pairs with feedback.
- Small group skills teaching using mannequins, e.g. taking a cervical smear.
- Practising EMQs/OSCEs with past questions and tutor feedback. See also Resources section below for books of example questions.
- Past students attending to give feedback to the group about their PLAB 2 exam experiences and the OSCE stations used.
- Small group discussions centring on various topics of interest to the PLAB, e.g. discussing case studies to look at ethical dilemmas.
- Involving students directly in sourcing information and teaching each other. This might be done by deciding on a topic relevant to the whole group, sub-sections of which are given to individual students who volunteer to read up about their sections and present to the rest of the group at the next meeting, e.g. type 2 diabetes.
- Role-play to practise communication skills, e.g. forming groups of three (where students act as doctor, patient and observer to feedback) to practise obtaining informed consent for an inguinal hernia repair.

The first five teaching formats listed above are most familiar or readily understood by the doctors from several countries that may be involved in a refugee group; thus they are most readily accepted. For PLAB 1, didactic teaching and practising EMQs with an expert are initially often prized above peer group learning. In preparation for the PLAB 2 OSCE, the doctors have often indicated that they value feedback from 'experts' only, discounting the value of feedback from peers.

When didactic teaching is used, the presentation should be as interactive as possible. Other learning methods are often more productive, certainly in terms of longer term retention of information and skills, but may need a little extra initial input to gain the confidence of the doctors. With this they are often enthusiastically received. An added advantage of peer-led learning skills development in the tutor-led study group is that the skills may be employed to improve learning capability at times when no tutor is available, e.g. in the peer-led discussion groups.

Evaluation and monitoring of study clubs

Funders will quite reasonably expect monitoring of the club's outcomes and evaluation is important for achieving quality. At the most basic level, monitoring should include a register and the collection of data on the progress of students through examinations and into jobs. Where possible, there should be fuller, more standard educational evaluation of individual seminars, club activities as a whole and learning needs and achievements of students. The register should be straightforward to achieve. Further than this, however, even following the exam progress of club members can be difficult. The problems are mainly in two areas: first, the members are usually keen to make use of every minute in the study club to take in medical knowledge and are not strongly motivated to fill in evaluation or progress questionnaires. This is a widespread problem across all medical education but it seems to be worse for this group who are so starved of educational opportunities which are particularly critical to their well-being.

Second, the group are extremely mobile and their social circumstances particularly fragile. They may drop in and out of the group according to whether they are experiencing problems with their families, housing, finances or if they are 'dispersed' away from London, as has recently been part of the Home Office's policy for asylum seekers. Even when not dispersed, they are often living in temporary homeless accommodation. This said, there should be a system for gathering and updating contact details where possible. Email is becoming increasingly important in this respect as it reaches people on the move and is becoming more universally accessible, at least in the larger cities. The Internet is often available at jobcentres and public libraries. The contact details could then be used to ensure a questionnaire periodically reaches all club members to check on progress and ask about their evaluation of club learning activities and their learning needs. The latter can contribute to formative evaluation of the club.

The merits and difficulties of the facilitated PLAB study group

The pros and cons can be looked at in terms of those applicable to the refugee doctors and those applicable to the tutor/facilitator. The following observations are based on study group tutors' experiences and feedback from students.

Living in a British city as a refugee attempting to pass an exam that allows you to work as an NHS doctor can be an incredibly isolating experience. Financial concerns, language barriers, access to relevant information, cultural differences and childcare difficulties are just some of the issues that compound this feeling of isolation. Attending a regular study group allows refugee doctors to meet other people in the same difficult situation from a range of overseas countries. This helps in the formation of friendships as well as affording the following additional benefits.

- The opportunity to share different cultural ideas from both experiences of work overseas and discussion about cultural issues applicable to the UK. This enables overseas doctors to understand that medicine is not universal in its approach but society specific; thus they appreciate the importance of learning about medicine as applied to the UK.
- A forum for sharing of knowledge with colleagues for mutual benefit. This includes feedback from other courses attended, PLAB exam experiences, sharing of information about future study course opportunities and teaching each other skills or knowledge from personal experience.
- Access to up-to-date information in specialist subjects from outside speakers with hands-on current experience of the NHS.
- A safe, friendly environment in which to practise clinical techniques and communication skills required for PLAB 2 with relevant feedback from a facilitator.

The limitations of PLAB study clubs currently, as fed back by refugee doctors, are the lack of resources for more outside speakers and more tutors to allow for smaller group teaching; a wider geographical spread of study groups to reduce travel time and costs; more time for longer study group teaching sessions.

The authors have found being teacher/facilitators for PLAB study groups a hugely rewarding experience and for them the pros far outweigh the cons. This is due to the overwhelming enthusiasm and hard work shown by refugee doctors who are very committed to learning, passing exams and practising as good doctors within the NHS. The difficulties are as follows.

- Large group size may limit the number of teaching techniques available for use and therefore also limit the subject material that can be taught.
- Financial restraints may limit resource availability, e.g. payments for outside speakers or money for equipment for teaching specific skills.
- The vast range between individual doctors in level of ability and previous clinical experience sometimes causes difficulty in gauging the depth of knowledge required in each teaching session.
- Educational concepts new to the refugee doctors, such as self-directed learning, can be difficult to integrate into teaching sessions due to the, often preferred, traditional teaching methods that refugee doctors have been used to in their home countries.
- The level of commitment needed to pass the PLAB exam makes the teaching of broader issues regarding healthcare in the UK more difficult (as students,

understandably, are less keen to learn about issues that will not directly affect their exam results).

- As refugee doctors are often isolated, they may seek advice about personal issues from a trusted study club facilitator. These issues may include financial problems, exam failures, social problems and personal health problems. These can be difficult and sensitive areas to address and require some anticipation and awareness of the appropriate services to refer doctors on to.

Study group case studies

The Refugee Health Professionals Project, Waltham Forest PCT

In early 1998 Rada Daniell, a refugee development worker, made contact with refugee and overseas doctors in her local area of the Redbridge and Waltham Forest Health Authority. Rada herself had been a refugee from Macedonia and was well placed to appreciate the difficulties and challenges facing asylum seekers and refugees in the UK. She approached the health authority and medical advisor for money to start a refugee project and a trust fund was eventually allocated.

Initially a series of regular meetings with refugee doctors was held and priority needs identified. One of the main priority needs was a requirement to pass the IELTS (an exam in English competency that is a prerequisite to sitting the PLAB exam). Accordingly the trust fund was initially used to pay for English courses (local PLAB revision courses were also commissioned).

In 2000, following a successful bid for a Single Regeneration Budget to fund a programme, Health Ladder to Social Inclusion, the health authority agreed to support a larger venture, the Refugee Health Professionals Project. (The management of this venture later transferred to the Waltham Forest PCT.) Whipps Cross University Hospital and Southwark and Waltham Forest College were used as resources to develop further training for refugee doctors to facilitate them in passing the IELTS and PLAB exams.

Within the project, the need for a PLAB study group was identified and subsequently one commenced in 2001 under the facilitation of Dr Geoff Norris, a local part-time GP and primary care tutor. The study club is open to local overseas doctors, whether refugee or otherwise. Doctors attend from all over the world, including Russia, Uzbekistan, Iran, Iraq, Pakistan, India, Congo, Afghanistan, Ukraine, Nigeria, Ghana and Madagascar. Immigration status is checked by the project administrator and then identification is provided for the doctors to enable them to use the educational resources of local hospital postgraduate education centres. Additionally, the local health authority has made available the resources of their library, including access to the Internet, as well as relevant textbooks to prepare for the PLAB exams. The facilitator has also invested allocated funds in reference books and anatomical mannequins to assist students in their preparation for the exam.

The study club is now starting to see a steady number of doctors obtain PLAB 1 and 2 and progress in their new NHS careers.

It is noteworthy that the establishment, progress and continuing viability of this study club have depended on the support of enthusiasts such as the manager and administrator of the Refugee Health Professionals Project as well as the study club facilitator Dr Norris, backed by the continuing financial support of the local primary care trusts.

East London Study Club

A group of refugee doctors in east London approached Queen Mary's College, University of London for support in setting up a club for studying and mutual support. This started in 1997, facilitated by Dr Sheila Cheeroth, a local GP in Tower Hamlets, supported by the college and the health authority (East London and City HA).

Since 1997, the study club has continued to meet for two hours on a weekly basis. During this time the Department of General Practice and Primary Care at Queen Mary's has developed a refugee doctor's programme which, as well as the weekly study club, now incorporates formal PLAB 1 and 2 study courses and a clinical attachment programme.

The study club is open to all who are interested. It is made up of approximately 30–40 students each week with some students leaving once they pass their exams and other new students joining. There is usually a large core of students who stay with the group for many months, even a year. The students come from all over London. A recent questionnaire handed out to study club students revealed further demographic details. Ages in the group range between 25 and 37 years. The students originate from the Middle East, Africa, Asia, Eastern Europe and South America. The dates that each of the students originally arrived in the UK range between 1997 and November 2002. Of the students who completed the questionnaire, just over 80% are unemployed. The three students who are employed work as a research fellow, OT assistant and locum phlebotomist respectively. The period of time since the students actually worked as doctors ranges between three months and five years. Their chosen areas of medical specialisation include general practice, general medicine, radiology, psychiatry, rheumatology, pathology and general surgery. All the students have passed their IELTS exam and 60% have passed PLAB 1.

At other times the make-up of the group has been quite different and this reflects the difficulty of addressing the breadth of needs of the entire potential group. In the last year there has been a growing dominance in the teaching of PLAB 2, reflecting the increasing proportion of the group who are preparing for PLAB 2 (the OSCE). This partly reflects the strengths of the teacher (JS), the availability of clinical skills teaching equipment not previously accessible and the difficulty in getting specialist teachers for PLAB 1 topics. In the past we have worked in a traditional lecture theatre, with no access to equipment and more access to specialist speakers, so the teaching and therefore the group were more PLAB 1 oriented. This illustrates the flexibility that is useful in running a study club, but also the limitations of resource that prevent it addressing all needs.

Included in the appendix to this chapter is a copy of our study club's most recent timetable as an example of the topics covered. This timetable is repeated in roughly the same form three times a year and is updated regularly on our website so that students have ample time for preparation and planning if required. Prior to having a set timetable, seminar topics were decided in a more informal way from week to week, depending on student suggestions. This proved to be more stressful for the facilitator in terms of planning, did not allow students sufficient time for preparation and did not give the facilitator or the students an opportunity to reflect on longer term goals and learning objectives.

Resources

Access to a basic range of up-to-date medical textbooks is necessary. Additionally, the following resources are especially pertinent to PLAB preparation.

- www.gmc-uk.org (contains a suggested syllabus of topics for the exam)
- www.plabmaster.co.uk (this site has information about past exam questions and tips on exam technique)
- Coales U (2000) *PLAB 1000 Extended Matching Questions*. Royal Society of Medicine Press, London.
- Coales U (2001) *100 Objective Structured Clinical Examinations*. Royal Society of Medicine Press, London.
- Feather A, Dimizio P, Field B, *et al.* (2001) *EMQs for Medical Students, Vols 1 and 2*. Pastest, Cheshire.
- Feather A, Visvanathan R, Lumley JSP, *et al.* (1999) *OSCEs for Medical Undergraduates*, Vols 1 and 2. Pastest, Cheshire.
- Dornan T and O'Neill P (2000) *Core Clinical Skills for OSCEs in Medicine*. Churchill Livingstone, London.
- Lloyd M and Bor R (2002) *Communication Skills for Medicine*. Churchill Livingstone, London.
- Gleadle J (2003) *History and Examination at a Glance*. Blackwell Science, Oxford.
- Audio Visual Production Unit. *Clinical Examinations, Series 1 and 2* (videos). Medical and Dental Media Resources, St Bartholomew's and Royal London School of Medicine and Dentistry, London.

Appendix: study club timetable for winter term 2003

Please see website to keep up to date with any changes.

4th September An introduction to the principles of medical ethics (SC)	PLAB 2 exam feedback from a previous student OR EMQs for PLAB 1 (JS)
11th September Chest X-ray Teaching (Dr Sahdev, consultant radiologist)	Resp EMQ and OSCE practice combined (SC)
18th September HRT tutorial (JS) OR EMQs for PLAB 1 (SC)	ENT examination and essential ENT for the newly qualified doctor (Mr Persaud)
25th September How to take a BP (practical session) (JS and SC)	Obtaining informed consent (JS) OR EMQs for PLAB 1 (SC)
2nd October Examination of the thyroid gland and the hand (JS)	
9th October Cranial nerve examination (JS)	Taking a neurological history with case studies (JS) OR Neurological EMQs for PLAB 1 (SC)
16th October Taking a GI history with case studies (JS)	Rectal examination (practical session) (JS) OR Practise GI EMQs for PLAB 1 (SC)
23rd October The management of perioperative problems in surgical patients (Mr Power, Specialist Registrar, General Surgery)	
30th October An introduction to depression/anxiety and assessing suicide risk (JS)	
6th November Taking a cervical smear (practical session) and interpretation and explanation of smear results (JS and SC)	

13th November A practical session on inhalers and PEFR meters (Glenda Esmond, Nurse Lecturer)	
20th November Telephone consultations and assessment of acute paediatric cases (JS)	Assessing the unconscious patient (Dr Tim Bell, A&E consultant)
27th November Eye examination and retinal pathology (Mr Westcott)	Taking a cardiovascular history with case studies. EMQs in cardiology for PLAB 1
4th December The principles of breaking bad news (JS)	Obs & Gynae history taking with case studies (JS) OR EMQs in Obs & Gynae problems for PLAB 1 (SC)
11th December Assessing the mini mental test score (JS)	Feedback session
18th December Christmas quiz and party	

JS – Dr Jo Scrivens
SC – Dr Sheila Cheeroth

CHAPTER 9

Clinical attachments in primary and secondary care

Yong-Lok Ong and Penny Trafford

Introduction

The Report of the Working Group on Refugee Doctors and Dentists, convened by AGMETS (Advisory Group on Medical and Dental Education Training and Staffing) and published by the Department of Health in 2000,[1] stated that one of the most beneficial ways of helping refugee doctors trying to re-establish their careers in the UK is by clinical attachments. This process is a well-used pathway undertaken by numerous overseas doctors seeking medical employment. There is, however, some anxiety about the varying quality of clinical attachments and much discussion of the difficulties refugee and overseas doctors face in securing an attachment and the reasons for these. There is little or no argument about the advantages for refugee and overseas doctors undertaking attachments in terms of familiarising overseas qualified doctors with NHS practice and culture and as a means of obtaining a UK consultant and GP reference, essential for getting a job. The ultimate value is the benefit to patient care as overseas qualified doctors equipped with a better understanding of the NHS will provide a higher quality service for patients.

Individual clinical attachments

Traditional attachments have been organised on an individual basis by the doctors themselves. This has largely depended on having an NHS consultant contact. Refugee doctors when compared to overseas doctors are at a disadvantage as many do not have the necessary introduction due to the circumstances of their arrival in this country. To compound the situation, there is a growing impression that the number of clinical attachments for overseas qualified doctors is failing to keep pace with demand and the number of attachments available may be declining. Many consultants are reluctant to take on any more attachments due to the large increase of undergraduate medical placements and the fear that taking on attachments may dilute the clinical experience and teaching time for those already in training. Refugee doctors who are successful in gaining attachments achieve them through persistence and luck, a winning ticket in the lottery of a system governed essentially by chance.

The fortunate doctors who obtain clinical attachments have hopefully received some career guidance beforehand on the appropriate timing to take on an attachment and the specialty to do it in.

Timing

Clinical attachments are thought to be most helpful at the pre-PLAB 2 stage as a means of preparing doctors for the examination, in particular the OSCE, and at the post-PLAB stage when doctors are job ready, to improve chances of making the shortlist and to equip them for job interviews. There is little possibility of experiencing two attachments and refugee doctors need guidance on the best time to apply for attachments according to individual needs. Refugee doctors who have been out of medicine for several years may benefit from attachments to bring their knowledge up to date for the PLAB 2 examination.

Specialty

Refugee doctors tend to choose specialties for attachments in which they have had experience and hope to pursue their careers. However, they may have less chance of training opportunities in the oversubscribed specialties of surgery, internal medicine and obstetrics and gynaecology. Guidance in the direction of specialties with training opportunities may prove to be a more beneficial use of attachments.

Primary care attachments

Few attachments in primary care are organised and where there are local contacts, the refugee doctors have short placements of a few weeks. Most refugee doctors do not realise the value of having an attachment in general practice even if they wish to pursue a career in primary care. This is because they are familiar with the consultant/acute sector model both in terms of their experience and their view that only consultants can give appropriate references. Overseas doctors have so little understanding of primary care and the differences from hospital medicine that they do not realise that without a GP attachment and hence without some experience of UK general practice, they are unlikely to be successful in GP VTS interviews. However, due to the one-to-one consultations in primary care and the service commitment, GPs can only give a longer and educationally appropriate attachment if there are financial resources allowing them to fund locums whilst they do the teaching. We recommend reimbursement at the same level as received for undergraduate teaching. Without registration or being on the supplementary lists of the PCTs, these overseas doctors have to function within primary care like a senior medical student.

They have little control over the length and quality of clinical attachments in a system that relies on goodwill. Anecdotal evidence gathered from refugee doctors shows a marked variation in both these areas.

Length

The ideal length of hospital-based clinical attachments agreed by educational supervisors is 2–4 months and for GP experience, six weeks in primary care and six weeks in one hospital job. Refugee doctors have reported a range of attachments from two weeks to eight months.

Quality

Standards of clinical attachments can vary enormously across NHS trusts and within primary care and they are often unstructured with a lack of clear aims and objectives for the attached doctors. There is usually no system for appraisal. Refugee doctors have reported being neglected during attachments and at times even rejected by members of the multidisciplinary team as an unnecessary demand on the team's time. They also often feel strongly that being an observer leads to little new learning of professional skills. In attachments where refugee doctors have been given the opportunity to perform the clinical duties of medical students, feedback has been more positive. The best experiences reported are from attachments where supervising doctors take personal interest in creating programmes for refugee doctors as part of their teams with supervised duties covered by medical indemnity.

Despite the helpful publication by the BMA of guidelines for clinical attachments,[2] there is still a great deal of variation between each individual attachment. This does not help refugee doctors and it is no wonder that many do not feel they have a good understanding of the NHS, particularly after a poor experience. Many are starting to think that the main purpose of clinical attachments is to obtain a local reference which credits them as being 'punctual and reliable' with 'fair to good clinical knowledge'. In trying to address some of these difficulties, the London Deanery has developed projects for refugee doctors in hospital medicine and general practice. These projects are described in detail in the rest of the chapter.

Pan-London Clinical Attachment Scheme

With funding received from the Department of Health (Refugee Health Professionals Steering Group) as part of the first phase of refugee health professional projects, a pan-London clinical attachment scheme for refugee doctors intent on pursing a career in hospital medicine was set up. A steering committee composed of clinical tutors, postgraduate deans and a refugee doctor met to develop the structure of the scheme. With knowledge of the difficulties faced by refugee doctors, the scheme was designed to offer the following features.

- Attachments for cohorts of 5–6 job-ready doctors in each participating trust. The cohorts were intended to provide group support for participating doctors and make best use of the trainers' time.
- A core curriculum defined by the steering committee, delivered to each cohort and supervised by a refugee project tutor on each site.
- Exposure to more than one specialty during the attachment.
- An evaluation by both tutors and refugee doctors of the value of the course and the usefulness of the structure agreed.
- Assessment in terms of the number of participating doctors who subsequently obtained medical jobs in open competition.
- Exploration of the factors which appeared to contribute to success or otherwise of refugee doctors in obtaining jobs.
- The length of the attachments would be for three months.

Over the course of three meetings, the steering committee agreed a core curriculum drawing from experience of members of the committee and from a model used for a pre-employment programme in Australia.[3] The curriculum was validated informally by asking the views of a range of clinical tutors in different specialties (Box 9.1).

Box 9.1: Core curriculum items

1   Routine clinical items
- History-taking skills and physical examination (with consent when appropriate)
- Presentation of cases
- Good prescribing practice
- Blood and infection control, interpretation of blood results, ECGs and X-rays
- Treatment decisions, doctor–patient partnership, autonomy and consent

2   *Primary care experience*
- Sit in on surgeries
- Attend GP teaching events

3   *ATLS/ILS course*
- Dealt with centrally by the Deanery; however, trusts able to provide in-house training received the appropriate funding

4   *Educational and personal skills*
- Clinical audit project or teaching on audit skills
- How to be a member of the multidisciplinary/ward team
- Dealing with difficult patients
- Managing death and bereavement

The steering group also agreed the information to be collected on each participant, in order to identify factors that might have an impact on subsequent success in gaining jobs. This included personal details; the number of attempts at passing IELTS and PLAB; and support from family and organisations in the UK. Two optional self-rating questionnaires were also included. These were Beck's Depression Inventory (BDI), where a threshold score of 12/13 is seen as indicating at least mild depression, and the Post Traumatic Stress Disorder Symptom Scale (PTSD). For a clinical diagnosis of PTSD, DSMIVR criteria needed to be met as well as a symptom score of above 18. Ethical committee approval was obtained.

All acute hospital trusts in London were invited to participate and the first one in each of the five sectors of London to show interest was chosen. Each of these was then asked to appoint a refugee project tutor whose responsibility was to act as educational supervisor for its cohort and ensure the core curriculum would be delivered along with exposure to more than one specialty during the attachment. Invitations were sent out to those refugee doctors on the BMA and London Deanery databases who were known to have passed the requisite hurdles to be allowed to work as a registered medical practitioner in the UK. Doctors who had previously undertaken an old-style clinical attachment were not excluded as this scheme was felt to offer something different. Each doctor was interviewed and information was collected as set out above. At this interview doctors were given the choice of completing the BDI and PTSD scales. All complied.

Once the participants had been identified, an induction day was arranged for the entire group. This included talks on the structure of the NHS and its values; communication skills, including informal medical English; culturally sensitive ways of breaking bad news; and curriculum vitae writing. The doctors then went to their respective trusts for the next three months. Throughout the attachments regular contact was kept between the Deanery team, refugee doctors and tutors to provide immediate support for difficulties and queries. At the end of the attachments, closure meetings were held for doctors and tutors during which an evaluation of the scheme was carried out by means of questionnaires and open discussions.

The outcome of the scheme was encouraging. Over half of the doctors were appointed to jobs in open competition by eight months after the scheme had started. A detailed description and evaluation of the scheme has been published.[4] It was possible to identify what the participating refugee doctors and tutors found to be the more useful aspects of the clinical attachments. This included the cohort system, regular tutorials and supervision from the refugee project tutors, the core curriculum, the ability to write and get realistic references and exposure to more than one specialty. It was also possible to conclude that structured clinical attachments may be a useful step for refugee doctors towards employment in the NHS. Based on these findings, a more comprehensive clinical experience scheme for general practice has been developed. This is now described in full to give providers of potential schemes information on detailed planning.

Box 9.2: Vignette – Dr KA

Doctor aged 29.

Refugee from a war zone country where suffered severe personal losses.

Arrived in the UK in 1998. Granted indefinite leave to remain in 2001.

Stacked shelves in a supermarket, feeling unable to come to terms with major losses.

Passed IELTS and PLAB and decided to join Pan-London Clinical Attachment Scheme. Felt structure would rekindle career and being placed in a cohort would provide psychological support.

Completed attachment and was appointed to an SHO post in open competition. Continues to train in a rotational programme.

Describes clinical attachment as giving a fluency of medical learning which still stands in good stead. Feels being a doctor again has given dignity to the losses suffered.

Refugee Doctors Clinical Experience Scheme

Aims of the scheme

The GP Postgraduate Department of the London Deanery received funding under Phase 2 of the Department of Health Refugee Health Professionals Project for the Refugee Doctor Clinical Experience Scheme (CES). This project started in April 2003 with the first cohort of doctors and is continuing with the second cohort.

Box 9.3: Aims

- To develop clinical experience in general practice and the hospital environment
- To offer continuing language development post IELTS
- To provide IT skills
- To provide interview skills training
- To offer support in CV writing
- To develop a network of participating general practices and acute trusts

---

The goal of the clinical experience scheme is to enable refugee doctors to be successful in obtaining posts as SHOs or rotations on GP vocational training schemes and as GP registrars.

The steering group was set up with the collaborators of the bid and a representative from each of the five WDCs representing the five sectors of London. The group has been responsible for interviewing refugee GP tutors, a training day for the refugee GP tutors and interviewing the refugee doctors for the scheme. The Refugee Training and Advisory Service (RETAS) agreed to fund travel expenses and childcare arrangements for the refugee doctors.

The programme

The 12-week programme is divided into six weeks in primary care and six weeks in one hospital attachment. The aims and objectives for the GP attachments were clarified. The curriculum for the Phase 1 hospital attachment scheme was used for the hospital placements. Each refugee doctor is given an educational portfolio. The scheme includes a two-day induction course covering the structure of the NHS, clinical governance, the consultation and general practice.

Box 9.4: Programme

- Wk 1   Induction course 2 days
- Wk 2–7   GP attachment (5 sessions)
- Wk 8–13   Hospital attachment (4 sessions)
- Wk 8–13   IT course
- Wk 2–13   Half-day release

Box 9.5: Educational provision

- Education agreement between tutor and RD
- Tutorials one to one every week
- Education portfolio
- Audit during GP attachment
- Learning needs assessment at beginning
- Assessments and feedback after each attachment
- Language and medical course organisers facilitating half-day release
- IT training (6 modules)

A half-day release course is held during the 12 weeks of the primary and secondary care attachments. The course organisers for the half-day are GP educationalists and IELTS teachers working together. The programme covers communication skills, interview skills and CV writing and continuing professional development.

Refugee GP tutors

One of the aims of the programme is to build up the critical mass of GP practices who will teach and mentor refugee doctors in a primary care attachment. A half-day training for the tutors was held to discuss the problems for refugee doctors and the issues for teaching and learning.

General practitioners are unable to give the commitment to one-to-one teaching as required in this scheme without appropriate reimbursement as this considerably affects the workload of the practice. Therefore, the refugee GP tutors are paid an amount equivalent to that for teaching undergraduate medical students.

Criteria for inclusion of refugee doctors on the Clinical Experience Scheme

The criteria for inclusion of refugee doctors on the scheme were agreed as follows.

- Passed IELTS
- Refugee status/ELR/ILR

- Spouse of those with refugee status/ELR/ILR
- Those who have entered the EU with refugee status
- Preparing for PLAB 2 or post PLAB 2
- Those who are committed to a career in primary care
- Those who live within London Deanery and five London WDC boundaries.

All doctors accepted onto the Clinical Experience Scheme have a police check and health check and obtain associate membership of the MDU.

Following the six-week placements in the general practices and hospital departments, the GMC form 'Request for a report on the clinical attachment undertaken by doctor' was used to assess the refugee doctors. The refugee doctors and the hospital and general practice tutors also filled in a questionnaire in order for us to evaluate the scheme.

Results, outcomes and evaluation

The refugee doctors reported that as a result of the scheme they had increased confidence in clinical skills and English language in consultations. They also had a greater understanding of UK general practice and the roles of members of the primary healthcare team, felt more prepared for applying for posts and had developed CV and application form writing and interview preparation skills.

They found it frustrating being in an observer position and wanted to take a more active part within the clinical team. The IT course had a mixed response as many of our refugee doctors had good IT skills.

Twelve refugee doctors were in the first cohort (April to June 2003) and 24 refugee and overseas doctors are still completing the second cohort. At the present time 10 of the 27 post-PLAB 2 doctors have substantive posts for August 2003 or February 2004, nine of these on GP vocational training schemes.

A personal story by one refugee doctor

My journey to be a GP

'In order to prepare myself for the PLAB part 2 exam, I attended the PLAB study group at Postgraduate Centre for Refugee Doctors in Hendon. It was a very useful and interesting experience at the same time. First of all, the Director of the Centre, Dr Nayeem Azim, tried his best with his colleagues at the centre to keep our professional knowledge and skills up to date. They also helped us in preparing our CVs.

Moreover, the centre was very well equipped with all the modern equipment and instruments, which we need in our training sessions, e.g. sphygmomanometers, stethoscopes, ophthalmoscopes, otoscopes, peak flow meters, etc.

Besides, there are more than 20 manikins (dummies) of different shapes, we used to enhance our clinical skills and to practise different tasks, e.g. CPR (basic life support), chest examination, breast examination, IV cannulation, blood collection, suturing, catheterisation, rectal examination, vaginal examination, etc.

At the end of the course we had a mock test similar to the real PLAB test which included different objective structured clinical examination cases (history taking, counselling, clinical examination and clinical skills).

Due to this pleasant atmosphere I passed the PLAB part 2 test on my first try.

I then undertook a clinical attachment at Grovemead Health Centre as part of the GP Support Worker Scheme co-ordinated between the Postgraduate Centre for Refugee Doctors and Barnet Primary Care Trust. For the duration of the attachment I was involved in carrying out a primary health assessment on newly registered patients. At the same time I started to work as a lecturer (part time) at North Central London College, teaching and training overseas doctors who are preparing for the PLAB Part 2 examination.

I then applied for the Refugee Doctor Clinical Experience Scheme in north London. This involved up to 24 hours per week for 12 weeks (from April to June 2003), obtaining clinical experience in hospital and general practice, post IELTS language development and IT training. There was mandatory attendance at a half-day release (Tuesday pm) for group learning facilitated by Dr Penny Trafford, Dr Geoff Norris and Tony Fitzgerald (IELTS provider, Barnet College).

I spent the first six weeks at Rosemary Surgery under the supervision of Dr Madhvi Shah (my GP tutor) and the remaining six weeks with Dr Ian Pollock (consultant paediatrician) at Chase Farm Hospital.

It was a very useful and interesting scheme. It assisted me to improve and also to gain new knowledge on different issues which I needed before starting to work in the UK.

First of all, it helped me to have a good picture on the UK medical, legal and cultural traditions. It answered my questions on how the NHS works and what is the role of the UK general practitioners in it. I understood that general practice is an organisation and not a "doctor work only clinic". The GPs are self-employed people and they work among a multidisciplinary team composed of the practice manager, practice nurses, receptionists, health visitors, district nurses, etc.

I learnt that general practice involves teamwork and mutual respect of the skills and contributions of each colleague. Trust, good communication, being a team player and understanding who is responsible for each aspect of the patient's care are important in teamwork. I also learnt that listening to other people's viewpoints, dealing openly and supportively with problems, collaboration and maintaining professional relationships with patients are important factors to make a good team function well.

In addition, the scheme helped me to view new ways of thinking, especially in improving my consultation skills. Before, I was used to a doctor-centred questioning approach in the consultation (i.e. I interviewed the patient, interrogated him, then diagnosed and treated his illness), which is very valuable in emergency situations, like in managing a cardiac arrest condition, where it does not help to ask a patient about their feelings! Now I follow the patient-centred approach in consultation due to it improving patient satisfaction. I started to read books about the consultation, like the one written by Roger Neighbour, *The Inner Consultation*, and *The Consultation: an approach to teaching and learning* by Pendleton. In addition to the five checkpoints of the consultation mentioned by Neighbour, I liked his ideas of housekeeping (self-awareness of one's feelings at moments within and between consultations) and minimal cues (the verbal and non-verbal "physical signs" to the patient's inner world of thoughts and feeling). I also learnt from the Pendleton book his seven tasks of the consultation, especially the one concerning finding out the patient's ideas about the cause of symptoms, his concerns about what might happen, his expectations about what the GP might do and finally the effects of the problem on the patient and his psychosocial environment.

During my clinical attachment at Rosemary Surgery I did one medical audit about the effective monitoring of thyroid function in chronic thyroxine treatment.

The course organisers worked very hard throughout the course to meet our learning needs and solve our problems in order to help us to become autonomous practitioners and conform to the standards of good medical practice. The IELTS course organiser played a very important part in improving our language skills, especially during the role-play scenarios. He taught us to use open-ended rather than closed questions, so that the patient says more than "yes" and "no" and the information generated is more reliable than if it had been framed by the doctor's assumptions in asking a closed question.

I now know that being a GP or family doctor, as I like to refer to the job (consultant in family medicine, as my wife prefers), I will play a very important role in the NHS, as I will provide the primary care for a huge number of people of all ages, from the cradle to the grave, in the local area. Moreover,

I like to manage the patients thoroughly (holistic approach) as GPs do by looking at the physical, emotional, social, economic and spiritual aspects of the patient, because the illness may not be apparent at first or one set of symptoms may be masking the real problem.

Besides the benefits I mentioned above, the scheme helped me to develop my IT skills, especially PowerPoint software presentations, and finally improved my interview skills.

On 17 June 2003 I attended the interview for the refugee rotation in general practice held at the BMA. The panel were very friendly and competent. They welcomed me first, then they introduced themselves one by one and made me relax. The interview lasted 45 minutes and I did very well. After two days I received a letter from the London Deanery offering me a three-year place on the Chase Farm GP Training Scheme within the London Deanery. The rotation will start on 6 August 2003. I am now looking forward to starting my new job at Chase Farm Hospital.'

Husham Majid

Innovations and the way forward

Both projects illustrate a need for structured clinical attachments as the way forward for refugee doctors to achieve success in gaining medical employment. The factors considered useful by both doctors and tutors who have participated in the schemes are new to the concept of clinical attachments and include:

- centralised selection interviews to establish aims of attachments
- placements in cohorts of 5–6 doctors in hospital attachments
- a core curriculum
- additional supervision by an identified attachment tutor and supervising consultants. In GP attachments this has been refined to close educational supervision in a 1:1 relationship with the GP tutor
- exposure to more than one specialty in hospital-based medicine during attachment
- full six-week attachment in primary care and a hospital specialty attachment for refugee doctors intending to become GPs
- a generic induction programme augmented by trust-level induction
- regular contact between supervisors and tutors and doctors
- closure meetings between refugee doctors, tutors and supervisors to identify the next training stage for the refugee doctor.

There are also a number of themes running through these innovative interventions. Refugee doctors need psychological support as they are sensitive to perceived rejection during attachments. This is provided for by the doctors being placed in cohorts, giving extra supervision from tutors and during the induction courses. They need clear educational objectives throughout their attachments.

Appropriate selection of the refugee doctors is best done through centralised selection interviews carried out by deaneries (possibly in conjunction with participating trusts and NHS Professionals). The learning needs of refugee doctors are more appropriately met by having a core curriculum for essential learning and regular evaluations during attachments. The final evaluation determined at the closure meeting is probably the most important as it will highlight the next training stage.

Educationalists in primary and secondary care should plan clinical attachments together to capitalise on pooled resources and their expertise in their own clinical fields. Hospital-based attachments could usefully have a two-week full-time attachment with an established GP tutor, so that the overseas doctors have a real appreciation of primary care, rather than the limited exposure of sitting in on a few surgeries, as is frequently the case. Likewise, potential GPs could carry out their hospital-based attachments with a known supervising consultant to gain a similar high-quality experience. As a result, the quality of clinical attachments for refugee doctors will then improve greatly, ensuring a good educational and supportive experience.

References

1   Advisory Group on Medical and Dental Education Training and Staffing (2000) *Report of the Working Group on Refugee Doctors and Dentists.* Department of Health, London.

2   Cheeroth S and Berlin A (2001) *Guidelines for Overseas Qualified Doctors.* British Medical Association, London.

3   Sullivan EA, Wilcock S, Ardzejewska K and Slaytor K (2002) A pre-employment programme for overseas-trained doctors entering the Australian workforce, 1997–99. *Med Educ.* **36**(7): 614–21.

4   Ong YL and Gayen A (2003) Helping refugee doctors get their first jobs: the Pan-London Clinical Attachment Scheme. *Hosp Med.* **64**(8): 488–90.

CHAPTER 10

Refugee doctor GP VTS rotations

Patrick Kiernan and Penny Trafford

Introduction

Patrick Kiernan and Penny Trafford are GP principals in London and both work as medical educationalists. Patrick Kiernan is a course organiser at St Mary's GP Vocational Training Scheme and was instrumental in initiating the first UK GP training scheme for refugee doctors in November 2001. Penny Trafford is an associate director of postgraduate general practice, leading on refugee doctors, and has been encouraging the establishment of further training schemes for refugee doctors across London.

Background

Refugee doctors

There are few initiatives, nationally, that help refugee doctors to get back to work in substantive career posts. Most focus on providing support for preparing for the International English Language Testing System (IELTS) and the Professional and Linguistic Assessment Board (PLAB) tests. Both are routes required for registration to work in the NHS, but passing the tests is only the first hurdle.

The General Medical Council will grant these doctors limited registration status only as long as they are appointed to approved or substantive hospital SHO posts. The GMC is in the process of reviewing the rules around registration, but as this requires change in legislation, the changes are unlikely to be implemented before 2005.

Many cannot find jobs in the NHS in open competition with local graduates, especially in cities like London. Therefore, refugee doctors often leave London to get posts in less competitive areas of the UK. For some refugee doctors, particularly those with families, London often continues to be their base, as they undertake a series of six-month SHO posts around the UK. As a result, there are hundreds of refugee doctors in the UK who remain unemployed and on benefits, unable to work as doctors.

Health needs of London

Meanwhile the NHS has an acute shortage of GPs and *The NHS Plan* has set a target to increase the number of GPs by 2000 in England by March 2004. Nowhere is this shortage of GPs more evident than in inner-city areas within the capital.

London is home to a large number of refugees and meeting the health needs of this population is a challenge to London GPs. There are many innovative projects, which are frequently under-resourced and funded on short-term monies, attempting to meet this service need and many GPs are managing their best with interpreters, advocates or family members translating. The refugee doctors already living within London are a motivated group of professionals wanting to return to their careers, who can meet the health needs of those refugees living within our communities as they are often from similar communities, able to speak the same language and with an understanding of the culture.[1]

Training programmes for refugee doctors in London

It is clear from other refugee initiatives that a coherent training programme is needed for these doctors to enter general practice. A lot of educational support is required to help these doctors become job ready and be competitive in the jobseeker's market. There are few initiatives that help refugee doctors successfully gain places on GP training schemes.

The London Deanery has funding agreed for 29 refugee doctors to undertake GP VTS three-year rotations across London. The first cohort of doctors started in November 2001 at St Mary's Hospital NHS Trust and since then, other rotations have started at Chase Farm Hospital (Barnet and Chase Farm Hospitals NHS Trust) and Homerton Hospital NHS Trust. Nine posts are to be recruited for February 2004 (St Mary's second cohort and Whipps Cross University Hospital NHS Trust) and funding for another six places is allocated for August 2004 (Fig. 10.1).

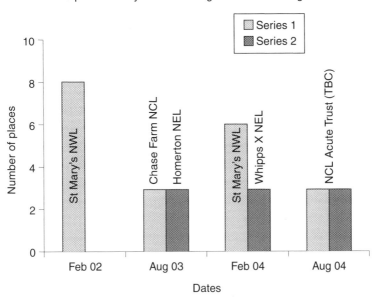

Figure 10.1 GP training places for refugee doctors in London.

St Mary's GP training scheme for refugee doctors

What follows is a description of the St Mary's scheme and the learning points that have arisen over the past two years.

The beginning of the scheme

In August 2001 Patrick Kiernan, as course organiser of the established St Mary's GP VTS, was approached by the Director of Public Health at the local health authority requesting help to put together a proposal for a GP training programme for refugee doctors. A sum of money had been identified and the DPH felt a bid for such a scheme might be well received at the Department of Health, if the project could be started and budget used within the financial year.

Within four weeks eight SHO posts had been identified with commitment from the hospital consultants. The SHO jobs were based at St Mary's and Central Middlesex hospitals, with a two-year hospital rotation, each job lasting six months, and included:

- paediatrics
- paediatric A & E
- adult A & E
- obstetrics and gynaecology
- care of the elderly
- psychiatry
- general medicine
- an ambulatory post of dermatology, genito-urinary medicine and palliative care.

The support and commitment from the consultants and GP trainers involved were extremely positive. In discussion, personal stories were told of parents or uncles and aunts who had come to this country as refugee doctors following the Second World War and who found it very difficult to get work and often had to fully retrain.

In costing the project, we went for maximum numbers within the available budget and opted for the posts not to have banding arrangements. The total cost per annum during the SHO years was £248K to include salaries, SHO training grants, course organiser payment and administration. If we had gone for banding arrangements, it would have nearly halved the number of doctors we were able to take onto the scheme.

The project received many excellent applications, many having experience of working in primary care in their own countries. Eight candidates were selected, four to start in November 2001 and four in February 2002.

Before starting the hospital posts, a two-week GP attachment was organised among the local training practices to provide an introduction and orientation to general practice.

Education and service provision

The SHO posts had established education agreements and training objectives, as well as three-way six-monthly appraisals with the relevant consultant and course organiser. Emphasis was placed on the importance of the induction training and gradual introduction to service delivery. It was felt that adequate learning and service delivery could be achieved within a full-time 40-hour contract, as well as gaining emergency cover experience within this time. We were concerned about doctors from a variety of cultural and training backgrounds, who were unfamiliar with the workings of the NHS, being 'thrown in at the deep end'. We were also concerned about placing these doctors into demanding and stressful out-of-hours night duty, very early on in the post, with the risk of not having adequate supervising cover.

A parallel weekly half-day release programme was set up which overlapped with the established GP VTS. This involved the first $1\frac{1}{2}$ hours with the course organiser, followed by a joint session with the established scheme with a visiting speaker. A short afternoon break then allowed for further integration.

Both schemes also attended the annual two-day residential. Further opportunities for integration existed as many of the postholders worked alongside GP SHOs in the established scheme.

The course organiser's main role was to hold the project together by acting as teacher, advocate and administrator, as well as liaising with consultant colleagues arranging rotations, promoting and publicising the project. The main educational challenge facing the course organiser was not only the bringing together of such a culturally diverse learning set through periods of change, but also orienting the group to working in NHS hospital posts.

During the two years of the scheme, there was variation in the educational supervision provided in each of the posts. This problem is not unique to refugee schemes and is continually being addressed by course organisers in established GP VTSs. However, such variation does present increased problems because of the need for greater supervision and support for these doctors. Educational agreements, regular appraisal meetings, with discussion and support in the VTS weekly half-day programme helped to address this issue.

Topics covered in the St Mary's half-day release programme for refugee doctors are listed in Box 10.1.

Box 10.1: Topics for half-day release for refugee doctors

- Understanding the NHS, primary and secondary care
- Different models of training received in different countries and how they translated to NHS posts
- Negotiation skills to navigate their way through the NHS
- Understanding of and working with multidisciplinary teams
- Reflection on clinical and organisational scenarios
- How to construct appropriate clinical management plans
- Chronic disease management
- Partnership with patients
- Communication skills
- Overcoming fears and asserting oneself appropriately

Refugee doctors appointed to the scheme

The refugee doctors are from a variety of countries including Iraq, Afghanistan, Croatia and Somalia. From an early stage, it was apparent that these doctors were bringing added value to the posts. This included their maturity, established clinical knowledge and skills, e.g. previous work in their own countries in primary care, paediatrics, obstetrics and gynaecology. One member had worked as a consultant general physician in Croatia for five years. In their SHO jobs, they were also translators and advocates to the multicultural patient community of west London.

They committed themselves wholeheartedly to the available learning opportunities and feedback from appraisals (using a GMC structured proforma) and identified a rapid assimilation into the culture of the NHS as they moved through the SHO posts. They attended GP deanery-led courses from an early stage to familiarise themselves as much as possible with general practice training. Within 12 months of starting they were able to move from limited to full GMC registration, as they were working in substantive NHS posts. They all expressed a strong enthusiasm for working in London with inner-city communities.

Evaluation of the scheme

A mid-term evaluation took place in October 2002 under the guidance of the Director of Public Health. Strengths and areas for improvement were identified.

Strengths

The scheme was seen by the refugee doctors as a great opportunity for training in varied specialties, providing a rapid and supportive pathway, post PLAB, of entry to a GP training programme. The posts were viewed as not too stressful or pressurised, because of the reduced out-of-hours commitment, and were seen as family friendly. The scheme offered continuity and security over two years, which was extremely important to the doctors, having come from positions of great insecurity. They valued the opportunities for integration with the established GP VTS and appreciated the understanding and support of colleagues and consultants who recognised that they brought with them different skills and experience. They recognised the importance of a supportive refugee group with commonality of experiences and valued being able to work in London close to family and friends.

Problems faced and areas for improvement

It was felt that the induction period needed improving and the consultants should make their departments more aware of the postholder, to achieve greater integration. The educational and service agreement needed to be implemented early in the job (recognising that this had to be initiated both by the postholder as well as consultant). The job responsibilities of the refugee doctor required clarification in some of the posts. It was important to ensure that the postholder had clearly defined responsibilities, particularly around inpatient ward work.

Stigmatisation of post and postholder tended to occur, as they were supernumerary posts and carried no manpower approval.

The ambulatory post was first set up incorporating time in general practice. However, this was difficult to sustain as the postholders were unable to issue prescriptions because of their limited registration status. Furthermore, a GP training grant had not been incorporated into the original budget proposal.

There was a need for regular monitoring of the posts due to the variation in educational supervision. The low salary caused hardship and, as a consequence, the introduction of a minimum banding arrangement for the posts is being explored.

Two postholders resigned from the scheme at six and 12 months for personal reasons. This caused minimum disruption as it allowed an additional two refugee doctors to be recruited through the BMA refugee doctor database and the outgoing doctors were a step closer to full GMC registration.

Due to lack of availability of GP registrar posts within the St Mary's established GP VTS, they could not be offered at the outset of the scheme, so the doctors were only appointed to the two years in SHO posts. The second cohort of doctors, starting February 2004, are to be appointed for three years to include a GP registrar post and this scheme will be fully evaluated once again.

Outcome

The SHO component of the scheme ends in January 2004 and six of the eight doctors, who are eligible, will be taking up their full-time GP registrar posts, following successful appointments through the GP deanery recruitment and selection process.

Comments from refugee doctors

'I feel honoured to have been part of this scheme and have learnt so much in our weekly group about practising as a GP in this country.'

'After two years working as a ward aide and a translator since leaving my country, this scheme rebuilt my confidence and commitment to becoming a "real" doctor again.'

'It was a great opportunity for me to be in medicine again after a few years' pause. As with every pilot scheme there were a few problems and misunderstandings but overall it was very successful.'

'Good choice of hospital posts gave me the experience I need for general practice. Very useful every week meeting with other refugee doctors in the group to discuss our specific problems.'

Refugee doctors: attributes and areas of difficulty

Attributes of refugee doctors

The motivation and commitment of refugee doctors are evident to all those who have worked with them in the classroom, study clubs and group situations, seeing these doctors progress through the pathway to registration and then into substantive posts. They bring to the UK their clinical skills and experience from their countries of origin and often speak three but usually more languages, so can act as interpreters, translators and advocates. The positive attributes of refugee doctors are listed in Box 10.2.

Box 10.2: Positive attributes of refugee doctors

- Motivation
- Enthusiasm
- Commitment
- Maturity
- Experience
- Specific clinical skills from previous experience
- Interpreters/translators
- Advocates

Areas of difficulty for refugee doctors

By the time these doctors are ready to undertake GP training, some are settled within communities and with their families. Others are still living with uncertainty about their circumstances in this country or about their families back home. Whatever their situation, whilst wishing to remain where they may have settled, the difficulties and pressures around obtaining a substantive post make them willing to travel to any part of the UK. Having got through the IELTS and PLAB, it can seem that this last hurdle of getting a job is insurmountable.

Doctors from Iran, Iraq and Afghanistan (in 2003 the predominant countries for refugee doctors coming to the UK) are allocated to posts in their own countries without interviews so there is a lack of understanding about the process of application and interviews and hence anxiety about the unfamiliar procedure. The ability to 'sell oneself' and clearly state one's strengths (and weaknesses) does not come easily, as well as being difficult for many whose self-esteem has been lowered through their recent experiences.

Refugee doctors are frequently not successful at GP VTS interviews because they have little understanding of primary care in the UK. Although their CVs may have reference to general practice in their own countries, this is often very different from UK general practice, e.g. they refer to rural clinic settings or general medicine departments in hospitals. Refugee doctors usually do a hospital clinical attachment in the UK, but often do not realise they would benefit from a general practice clinical attachment for a career as a GP. In order to be successful in interviews for GP training, they need, in particular, an appreciation of the structure of the NHS, an understanding of general practice and teamwork, an ability to reflect on clinical cases and to discuss and reflect on clinical scenarios.

The areas of difficulty in substantive posts have been highlighted in the discussion of the St Mary's scheme and are summarised in Box 10.3.

Box 10.3: Areas of difficulty for refugee doctors

In applications

- Do not understand the process
- Need help with writing CVs and application forms
- Little or no experience of interviews in their own country
- Not used to 'selling themselves'
- Little understanding of primary care

In starting a substantive, supernumerary post

- Fear
- Lack of assertiveness
- Time required to make cultural shift
- Styles of communication
- Different models of training received in different countries
- Appropriate induction period
- Integration into hospital department
- Stigmatisation of post and postholder

Selection and recruitment

Criteria for selection of refugee doctors

The eligibility criteria for the refugee doctor GP VTS must be owned by all responsible for funding the schemes: the PCTs, strategic health authorities, WDCs and the deanery. Tension has arisen between trying to be inclusive in the criteria (hence helping refugee doctors to progress along the pathway back to medicine as quickly as possible) and avoiding the investment of resources in individual doctors who could possibly be returned home. Therefore, after much consideration, asylum seekers who have the right to work are excluded from applying to the GP VTS scheme.

The PCTs and WDCs were particularly concerned that budgets allocated should be used within their sector. City and Hackney PCT won a bid from the Neighbourhood Renewal Fund and it was felt important that this was used for refugee doctors living in Hackney. This led to a discussion around settled refugee doctors in localities having priority of places. However, finally, it was agreed that the best candidates should get the posts, as in any other GP VTS rotation. Retention of refugee doctors within a sector is more likely to occur if, on completion of GP training, the PCTs are proactive in organising suitable GP posts.

Doctors exempt from taking the PLAB exam were precluded from applying to the scheme. Exemption from the PLAB largely occurs because of specialist experience and in order to progress in that specialty, the RCGP does not sponsor these doctors on the senior doctor route. Secondly, exemption from the PLAB means the doctors have not had the difficulties of the IELTS/PLAB route, which is part of the justification for the positive action in setting up the refugee doctor GP VTS.

Box 10.4: Eligibility criteria for applicants

- Refugee doctors with refugee status, indefinite leave to remain or having gained British citizenship
- Exceptional leave to remain or humanitarian status
- To have remained ordinarily resident in the UK since status recognised
- Family reunion: a spouse of someone with refugee status, the spouse having been resident in the UK for one year
- Passed PLAB 2 (doctors with PLAB exemption not accepted)
- Able to secure limited registration with the GMC

Advertising

All the refugee doctor GP VTS rotations have been funded on non-recurring monies and usually the funding is agreed at the last minute! The rotations are also regarded initially as projects, subject to appropriate evaluations. It is hoped that following satisfactory outcomes, recurring funding will be secured to support subsequent cohorts of trainees. This has already been achieved at the St Mary's scheme, funded by the North West London WDC.

The BMA database for refugee doctors is now widely known and used both by refugee doctors and statutory and voluntary organisations. They are willing and efficient in sending out advertisements when requested and the network of participants is effective. Therefore, in recent adverts we have chosen not to use the *BMJ* but to use the BMA database.

Equal opportunities (EO) must be considered. In order for adverts for refugee doctors not to breach EO legislation, it must be clear that positive action is occurring, not positive discrimination. Advice was sought from the Human Resources Department of the London Deanery, the five WDCs in London and the Commission for Racial Equality which advised us:

'The Race Relations Act makes racial discrimination unlawful except in certain clearly specified circumstances:

- When an organisation is taking positive action to encourage people from a certain racial group to apply for a job or training because they are underrepresented in the organisation or at certain job levels [ss 35–38].

    Note: Section 37 of the Race Relations Act says that employers may restrict training for certain kinds of work to people from a particular ethnic group when they are underrepresented within the organisation or at certain job levels. Section 35 says that making arrangements to meet the special needs of people from a particular racial group in education, training, welfare or any ancillary benefits is not unlawful.

Publishers should ask employers and other advertisers who claim exemption for their advertisements under the Race Relations Act to quote the relevant section of the Act, and provide any other information the publishers may need to satisfy themselves that the advertisements are lawful. The text of an advertisement should also make it clear to readers why the exception applies to the job.'

The following clause is therefore included in the deanery adverts for the refugee doctor GP VTS:

'This advert is exempt from the Race Relations Act (see sections 35 and 37). Refugee doctors are underrepresented as GPs and arrangements are being made to meet the special needs of refugee patients.'

Recruitment

Although it is accepted that there is positive action to help refugee doctors obtain GP VTS posts, it is also important that these doctors are accepted as equals with other GP trainees in SHO and GPR posts. Therefore the same selection and recruitment procedure is used for refugee doctors as for other applicants within the London Deanery.

However, in looking critically at the procedures normally in place, we have taken certain steps to make the recruitment process more appropriate to overseas and refugee doctors.

Application pack

The deanery pack for all applicants was rewritten and made inclusive. We reviewed:

- the eligibility criteria
- the person specification for screening
- requests for documentation
- EO form
- the language used in the application form, which was unnecessarily difficult
- the structured reference form (different form used based on GMC clinical attachment reference form to accommodate refugee doctor's situation).

Training the interview panel

Refugee doctors have expressed their sense of frustration and feelings of being devalued, by not being given time in interview to explain their clinical experience in their own country. They also frequently do not get asked about the studying they have been doing for IELTS and PLAB or their UK clinical attachments. Some may be uncomfortable when speaking about their personal experiences of loss, and yet feel they should do so. Refugee doctors are also at a disadvantage because of their career gap. The interview is often in their third language, which makes it more difficult to express their ideas and opinions.

Therefore the interview panel is told before interview:

- to give more time for each interview
- to allow the applicant more time to express himself or herself in English
- that the fact that all applicants have a career gap is not a problem in itself
- to help the refugee doctor settle into the interview, questions should be asked about their medical experience in their own country and/or clinical attachments.

Posts

The SHO training posts for refugee doctors are supernumerary, i.e. do not have manpower approval as there are constraints on expansion of SHO training posts. In protecting these posts for refugee doctors, because of equal opportunities legislation, they must also be supernumerary. We have also had discussions about giving overseas doctors access to these posts. However, about 150 of the 600 or so applications received by the deanery every six months for GP VTS places are from overseas doctors. These doctors are choosing to come to this country for their own reasons and are not in the position of being forced to leave their countries of origin, as with refugee doctors.

Selecting the posts

The posts must be appropriate to the educational needs of the refugee doctors. Certain principles have been adopted by the London Deanery in tailoring the new refugee doctor GP VT schemes.

- A medical post is included in the rotation and this is best done in Care of the Elderly as there are usually no similar posts in the countries of origin of the refugee doctors.
- A longer period in primary care (18 months rather than 12 months) is often appropriate.
- The extra six months in general practice may be on a part-time basis, giving time to do work in other relevant specialties through secondments.
- The St Mary's scheme included the oncall commitment within a 40-hour contract, with enough in-hours emergency cover experience during the day.
- There needs to be flexibility to meet the individual educational needs.
- There must be enhanced educational support and mentoring.

Integration versus segregation

Two models have been adopted within the London Deanery for refugee doctor GP VT schemes.

- The St Mary's scheme has similar but different posts and contracts from other GP SHOs and separate teaching for part of the GP half-day release.
- The more recently developed schemes (Chase Farm, Homerton and Whipps Cross Hospitals) have posts that are identical with the other GP SHOs in the departments, the same half-day release and a mentor who meets regularly (together and individually) with the refugee doctors.

We intend to use feedback and evaluation of the two models to compare and contrast and, we hope, improve all the schemes.

There are potential problems in integrating refugee doctors into the hospital departments and general practices. There are beliefs amongst some staff that medical education in some other countries is inferior to UK training. There may be disguised racism or issues around language proficiency. Where the posts are different, there may be misunderstanding about the roles and responsibilities of the refugee doctors. At the St Mary's scheme, this required explanation and support to avoid stigmatisation, isolation and sometimes bullying of the doctors. The importance of a good induction is emphasised, to include a full explanation to all staff of the role of the postholder, as well as continued supervision.

When the St Mary's scheme started, there were few organised clinical attachments for refugee doctors. However, in London there are now clinical attachment schemes which prepare refugee doctors for work in the NHS and primary care: for example, the Refugee Doctor Scheme at Queen Mary University of London (Barts and the London Department of Primary Care), and the London Deanery Postgraduate Department of General Practice Clinical Experience Scheme for Refugee Doctors. Both of these schemes include the topics covered in the St Mary's half-day release for the refugee doctors (see Box 10.1).

From the applications so far, we are finding that the doctors from these clinical attachment schemes are much better prepared for the interviews for general practice training and work in the NHS and are being more successful in interviews.

In discussion on the half-day release, refugee doctors can contribute to each other's learning from their varying experiences. However, sometimes their experience is so different that it can make joint learning with an established VTS difficult; for example, a Somalian doctor who has little experience of the care of the elderly because of reduced life expectancy in his country or a doctor from Iraq who has practised general medicine with access to very few investigations and drugs. At the St Mary's scheme, it was felt that the training needs and cultural diversity of such a group reinforced the need to provide a separate learning set.

Educational approval

All the refugee doctor GP training schemes are endorsed by the London Deanery GP Education Committee and selected on behalf of the Joint Committee on Postgraduate Training for General Practice (JCPTGP) as suitable for GP training. The JCPTGP requires one year of the SHO posts to be educationally approved for GP training in hospital departments. The other six months of SHO posts in the scheme can be in an ambulatory or innovative post. Therefore, in choosing the supernumerary posts, we make sure they are in departments that have received at least a 'B' rating in the HRC/RCGP hospital visit report.

The Registrar of the JCPTGP is fully informed about all the schemes and supernumerary posts and has worked with us in making sure we conformed to the above standards. The St Mary's posts have been given approval under equivalent experience and we are assured the JCPTGP will do the same for the newer schemes. In addition, the consultants involved in the St Mary's scheme agreed to submit the posts for specialty training approval.

Contract arrangements

In the St Mary's scheme we explored a model of holding the contracts with the health authority (subsequently the primary care trust), with honorary contracts held with hospitals. The salaries were also paid though the PCT.

The posts were sited across three different trusts and, therefore, the advantages of this arrangement included centralised management and recruitment services and clarity of funding arrangements. It was also seen as a first step towards PCTs being the conduit for funding for GP training during the SHO posts.

All the other refugee doctor GP VT schemes have the same contract and payment arrangements and the second St Mary's cohort of doctors will follow this pattern.

Funding and the future

Securing funding for these schemes has been difficult. The St Mary's scheme received project monies from a number of sources. Generally, it has to be raised through the Deanery, PCTs and WDCs.

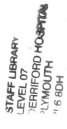

The GP Department of the London Deanery is currently supporting 12 or 18 months of the training from the GP Registrar budget. The other 18 months' financial support has to be found from the PCTs or WDCs.

City and Hackney PCT was successful in August 2002 in receiving funds from the Neighbourhood Renewal Fund to support some of the costs of the scheme based at the Homerton Hospital. City and Hackney is home to a large number of refugees. Given that around 5–6% of all refugees in the UK are settled in City and Hackney (Health of Londoners Report 1999) and using the BMA database for refugee doctors, the PCT assumed that as many as 50–60 medically trained refugees might live in their area. PCTs can find contributing to the cost of GP training prohibitive with their limited budgets.

Although WDCs and PCTs are striving to meet their workforce targets for 2004, they are understandably hesitant about contributing to the long-term rewards of paying for a refugee doctor's three-year general practice training when there are so many other calls on their limited funds. They are also seeking to obtain the monies required through bids, for example from the European

Refugee Fund, but with limited success. The view taken on the bids is that the usual training requirements for general practice should be found within existing NHS education budgets. After many discussions the WDCs in the north of London have all contributed some monies to the GP training of refugee doctors. None of the refugee doctor GP VT schemes have recurrent funding agreed.

Although the Department of Health has provided £500 000 in 2002 and 2003 to support bids made to the Refugee Health Professionals Steering Group, there is substantially more financial support needed from central resources to assist deaneries and WDCs in obtaining more GP training schemes for refugee doctors.

Reference

1   The GP Recruitment and Retention Report GLA June 2003.

CHAPTER 11

Developing the NHS workforce through innovative schemes

Sue Arnold and Neil Jackson

Introduction

One of the important features of modernising the NHS is the development of its workforce to meet the needs of the communities it serves. The kind of workforce required must be fit for practice and purpose, with the ability to work in multi-professional/multidisciplinary teams of healthcare professionals and capable of sustained learning and development.

Quality service provision of healthcare for patients relies upon a highly trained and motivated NHS workforce, within which refugee doctors as a valuable workforce resource must find their place.

This chapter will outline some specific principles which apply to developing and retaining the NHS workforce. Innovative schemes for developing the NHS workforce, which are currently being implemented for refugee doctors and other NHS staff, with the support of government and other funding streams, will also be described.

The principles of retaining and developing the NHS workforce[1]

Although the recruitment of healthcare professionals is crucial to the NHS as an employer in terms of adequate numbers and skill mix across various professional groups, so too is the retention and development of staff. This applies to both the primary and secondary care sectors of the NHS.

There are many principles which influence the retention and development of NHS staff. Some of these are employer or employee specific and some are shared between employer and employee as summarised below.

Employer-specific principles

- Retaining and developing the right number of healthcare professionals with the right knowledge, skills and attitudes to deliver quality service provision for patients.
- Defining and implementing a value-based approach to challenge abusive and inappropriate behaviour in the workplace, such as prejudice, bullying and violence.
- Appropriate induction programmes for all new staff members.
- Planning staff development to underpin corporate and clinical governance.
- Having an appropriate performance management system within the employing organisation related to retention and development issues.
- Putting support systems in place to manage stress and to encourage reflection in daily working lives.
- Maintaining a concern for all employees at all levels in the employing organisation; recognising and developing potential in each staff member and developing leadership qualities when appropriate.
- Securing sufficient resources to ensure investment in staff development.

Employee-specific principles

- Staff loyalty and commitment to the employing organisation and the NHS as a whole.
- Quality of working life for staff, particularly during 'out-of-hours' service provision.
- Regular appraisal and feedback on performance to encourage personal and professional development.
- 'Family-friendly' policies within the employing organisation to support flexible working for mothers with young children, etc.
- Fair rates of pay for employees and incentive schemes where appropriate.

Shared principles

- Shared values, aims and objectives between employers and employees at all levels within the NHS employing organisation.
- Corporate responsibility for retaining and developing staff to include input at board level and throughout the organisation, including individual employees/employee representatives.

- Learning together across professional/disciplinary boundaries at organisational, team and individual healthcare professional levels.
- Maintaining an appropriate balance between personal and professional development and employability in the NHS, i.e. continuing professional development for healthcare professionals which links personal and professional development needs to the wider needs of the employing organisation and the NHS as a whole.

Innovative schemes to develop the NHS workforce

The Skills Escalator[2] underpins the NHS approach to developing exciting and innovative careers in the NHS. Work-based education and training programmes form a part of life-long learning to recruit and retain staff.

The Skills Escalator is also about attracting a wider range of people to work within the NHS by offering a variety of step-on and step-off points. Traditional entry points for registered professional staff will continue but they will be complemented by other entry routes such as conversion of qualifications gained overseas, to enable people currently either unemployed or underemployed back into the labour market. This includes refugee doctors and other healthcare professionals.

This offers the dual benefit of growing the NHS workforce whilst also tackling problems of longer term unemployment and social exclusion, which have such a high correlation with poor health. It will also give the NHS a workforce that is more representative of local communities and enable better service delivery.

However, innovative and creative work-based training programmes often have a resourcing implication for NHS organisations that are already overstretched. As a result, strategic alliances are made with partners from both the statutory and non-statutory sectors, bringing together the knowledge, experience and, most importantly, the funding to implement new programmes.

A number of initiatives for refugee doctors are taking place across the UK, usually led by NHS workforce development confederations and deaneries, often in collaboration with community refugee organisations. Multi-partnership working is often the key to accessing external funding streams.

Within the Learning and Personal Development Division at the Department of Health,[3] a team has been established to review the provision of training for health professionals who qualified abroad. This includes the provision of clinical attachments for doctors, induction periods and structured training programmes.

Specific work is being undertaken for refugees who are qualified health professionals. The department has funded training courses and advice services, which prepare refugee health professionals for registration and work in the NHS. Helpful contacts for refugee health professionals can be found in the Refugee Health Professionals' Contact Network at: www.doh.gov.uk/medicaltrainingintheuk. The department's guidance on refugee health professionals' training can be found in the document *Report of the Working Group on Refugee Doctors and Dentists* which is available at the same site.

Education and training programmes funded by the Department of Health

Over the last three years, the Department of Health's Refugee Health Professionals' Steering Group has provided support for a number of projects for refugee doctors across the UK.

West Midlands health authorities

A large collaboration between various health authorities and academic centres in the West Midlands to provide:

- identification of refugee doctors
- regional information pack
- access to medical libraries
- mentoring with the Refugee Education and Training Advisory Service (RETAS) and Warwick and Birmingham universities
- clinical attachments (before and after registration)
- IELTS training at Brasshouse Language Centre
- PLAB training at Warwick and Birmingham universities
- ongoing support.

Contact

Mrs Jo Thanki
Heart of Birmingham Teaching PCT
Bartholomew House
142 Hagley Road
Birmingham B16 9PA
Telephone: 0121 224 4795
Email: jo.thanki@hobtpct.nhs.uk

Redbridge and Waltham Forest Health Authority Refugee Health Professionals' Project

Communication and clinical skills training for PLAB Part 2 at Southwark College, and clinical skills training for PLAB Part 2 preparation at Whipps Cross University Hospital.

Contact

Kat Huxtable
Refugee Health Professionals' Project
WLL PCT
3rd Floor, Becketts House
2–14 Ilford Hill
Ilford IG1 2QX
Telephone: 020 8926 5180 or 020 8926 5221
Email: kat_huxtable@hotmail.com

Liverpool School of Tropical Medicine

Creation and implementation of a postgraduate diploma programme in European medicine, along with language support for IELTS, preparation for PLAB, careers advice, interview skills and a UK clinical reference.

Contact

Dr James Bunn
Course Director
Liverpool School of Tropical Medicine
Pembroke Place
Liverpool L3 5QA
Telephone: 0151 705 3205
Email: jegbunn@liv.ac.uk

Refugee Clinician Programme

Refugee doctors' training in Bristol and South West, covering all aspects of training including:

- language skills (for IELTS and PLAB)
- clinical attachments
- clinical training (for PLAB)
- interview and career advice.

Contact

Michelle Griffiths
Project Manager
Refugee Clinician Programme
ESOL Unit, City of Bristol College
Brunel Centre
Ashley-Down Road
Bristol BS7 9BU
Telephone: 0117 904 5034
Email: Michelle.Griffiths@cityofbristol.ac.uk

Pan-professional projects

The examples listed above are those programmes specifically for refugee doctors. However, the Department of Health has sponsored a number of other programmes – too many to list here – that are suitable for all refugee health-care professionals. For further information contact:

Jonathan Firth
Department of Health
Quarry House
Quarry Hill
Leeds LS2 7UE
Telephone: 0113 254 5699

London programmes for refugee doctors

More than 50% of refugee doctors currently registered with the BMA/Refugee Council database live within London. Consequently, there are a number of innovative programmes available for doctors living within the capital. The following list are examples and not exhaustive. Readers should contact the London NHS WDCs for an up-to-date list of available programmes.

This chapter outlines some of the existing schemes available at the time of writing. However, as with those sponsored by the Department of Health – and provided elsewhere within the UK – new programmes are being developed all the time and readers are invited to contact either their local NHS WDC or the London Deanery which will be able to provide advice on programmes available within their sector. A list of workforce development confederations may be located at: www.wdc.nhs.uk

At the London Deanery, contact either Dr Yong-Lok Ong (programmes within the acute sector) on 020 7692 3366 or Dr Penny Trafford (programmes within primary care) on 020 7692 3054.

Workforce development confederations can advise and work with trusts and other organisations to identify and secure funding to support refugee doctor programmes.

North West London NHS Workforce Development Confederation

- Refugees into Jobs – journal club, careers advice, colloquial English language tuition, support for travel, exam fees and childcare.
- Westminster PCT Journal Club – as above.
- Hillingdon Refugee Healthcare Professional Project – careers advice, support for travel, exam fees and childcare.
- West Middlesex University Hospital – refugee doctor adaptation programme (pre and post PLAB refugee doctors).
- North West London Hospitals – SHO equivalent refugee doctor programme (post PLAB refugee doctors).
- Stepping Stones – pathway into employment for (pre-PLAB) refugee doctors providing paid employment combined with clinical attachments at Brent PCT and Hillingdon Hospital.
- General practitioner vocational training scheme for refugee doctors (post PLAB).
- Library support and access to KA24 (Internet-based journal and textbook library).

Contact

Sue Arnold
Assistant Director Access and Development
North West London NHS Workforce Development Confederation
Brentford
Middlesex TW8 9LX
Telephone: 020 7756 2776
Email: sue.arnold@nwlwdc.nhs.uk

North Central London NHS Workforce Development Confederation

- PLAB preparation at the North Central London College.
- Three-month structured clinical experience programme offering six weeks within primary care and six weeks within the acute sector. Additional support with IT and communication skills provided.

- General practitioner vocational training scheme for refugee doctors (post PLAB) at Chase Farm Hospital.
- Supplementary IELTS support.

Contact

Jonathan Barnwell
Associate Programme Director
Haringey Teaching PCT
TPCT Programme Centre
St Ann's Hospital
St Ann's Road
London N15 3TH
Telephone: 020 8442 6007
Email: jonathan.barnwell@haringey.nhs.uk

North East London NHS Workforce Development Confederation

- Queen Mary's Refugee Doctors' Programme – PLAB 1 and 2 training, journal club, clinical attachments.
- Refugee Health Professionals' Project – advice, IELTS, PLAB 1 and 2, journal clubs, clinical attachments.
- General practitioner vocational training scheme for refugee doctors (post PLAB) at Whipps Cross and Homerton Hospitals.
- Praxis – advice and guidance.
- Three-month structured clinical experience programme offering six weeks within primary care and six weeks within the acute sector. Additional support with IT and communication skills provided.
- Cardiovascular health technician programme at Waltham Forest PCT – work-based training and employment for refugee healthcare professionals
- Barking and Newham journal club.
- Library support and access to KA24 (Internet-based journal and textbook library).

Contact

Diana Cliff
Refugee Health and Social Care Co-ordinator
North East London NHS Workforce Development Confederation
Aneurin Bevan House
81 Commercial Road
London E1 1RD
Telephone: 020 7655 6714
Email: diana.cliff@nelwdc.nhs.uk

South East London NHS Workforce Development Confederation

- IELTS and PLAB 1 provision at Southwark College.
- Journal club at St Thomas' Hospital.
- Clinical attachments at King's College University Hospital.
- Three-month structured clinical experience programme offering six weeks within primary care and six weeks within the acute sector. Additional support with IT and communication skills provided.

Contact

Sarah Coleby
Assistant Director of Workforce Development – Careers
South East London NHS Workforce Development Confederation
South Bank Technopark
90 London Road
London SE1 6LN
Telephone: 020 7593 0119
Email: sarah.coleby@selwdc.nhs.uk

South West London NHS Workforce Development Confederation

- Three-month structured clinical experience programme offering six weeks within primary care and six weeks within the acute sector. Additional support with IT and communication skills provided.
- General practitioner vocational training scheme for refugee doctors (post PLAB) at Epsom and St Helier Hospitals.
- IELTS provision at Kingston, Croydon and Nescot Colleges.
- Library support within trusts.
- Epsom and St Helier Hospitals – SHO supernumerary refugee doctor programme (post PLAB refugee doctors).

Contact

Sylvia Onyekwelu
Recruitment and Retention Manager
South East London NHS Workforce Development Confederation
41–47 Hartfield Road
Wimbledon
London SW19 3RG
Telephone: 020 8545 7120
Email: sylvia.onyekwelu@swlwdc.nhs.uk

References

1 Jackson N (2003) Work based learning and the retention and development of the NHS workforce. *Work based Learning in Primary Care*. **1**: 5–9.

2 Department of Health Learning and Personal Development Division website: www.doh.gov.uk/hrinthenhs/learning/section4b/skillsescalatorhomepage

3 Department of Health Learning and Personal Development Division website: www.doh.gov.uk/hrinthenhs/learning/section2a/overseashealthtraininghomepage

CHAPTER 12

Careers advice and mentoring

Angela Burnett and Sheila Cheeroth

Introduction

This section is written bearing in mind the enormous variety in what is already available in different areas of the UK for refugees and for refugee doctors in particular. Thus it aims to describe the fundamental frameworks of service provision rather than be prescriptive.

The aim is to provide a comprehensive integrated careers guidance service in collaboration with other agencies working in the local area. The agencies may include the Department of Health's postgraduate deaneries and employment and training organisations in the statutory and voluntary sectors. Consultation with the current providers and users of advice services usually reveals unmet need in the area of specialised advice by and for medical personnel. The specific aim of a medical careers advice service is to guide the refugee doctor through a jobsearch process with complex and alien legal and professional cultural aspects, the appreciation of which is key to success. The process includes GMC registration, accessing appropriate courses, obtaining clinical attachments, writing job applications and being interviewed for a first UK medical post. Mentoring focuses more on promoting an individual refugee doctor's personal and professional development within a longer term relationship with a single mentor.

How to set up and run a medical careers advice service

Careers advice team roles

Usually the generic services can provide advice on educational grants, employment and training rights and courses for English language and IT skills. There is variability amongst employment and training agencies in their capacity to assist with issues specifically affecting refugees. If there are gaps in this area, advice should be sought from refugee organisations such as the Refugee Education and Training Advisory Service (RETAS) and the Refugee Council (see Resources section at end of chapter) so this can be addressed. Referral pathways need to be put in place between the generic agencies and the medical careers advice service. Ideally this would include referral on from the careers advice service for those with need for psychological support, welfare assistance, immigration advice and other needs which sometimes come to light during medical careers counselling but are best handled by experts in other fields.

The medical careers advice and guidance service exists to provide one-to-one careers counselling offered by doctors in NHS practice. The service the authors provided at RETAS was managed within a general refugee careers advice service and was complementary to it. This was found to be a very supportive and productive framework for all advisors. Good provision for team communication is essential. The administration will need to manage recruitment and training of advisors, to run the appointments, to manage client records, to monitor, evaluate and control quality of the service and resolve issues arising on a day-to-day as well as longer term basis. Experience shows that some common problems arise repeatedly in advice sessions with clients (such as lack of medical CV writing skills, lack of skills in filling in a job application form and no previous interview experience). Common needs flagged up during the careers advice sessions can often be usefully and time/cost-effectively addressed in a programme of workshops provided by the service.

Physical environment

It is vital that the service is run from a site readily accessible to public transport, bearing in mind the client group is usually without private transport.

It is essential that the environment affords privacy and a degree of comfort to facilitate a relaxed discussion where the refugee doctor feels he or she can be open about problems and fears. Many have been used to self-sufficiency and success and find dependence and unemployment distressing and shameful.

Advice centre resources

Essential

- Careers guides such as the very readable and useful *So You Want to Be a Brain Surgeon?*.[1]
- Up-to-date authoritative literature on training pathways and opportunities in the different specialty areas should be obtained from the Royal Colleges of

the different specialties – a list of the colleges can be found in RETAS handbook.[2] This information changes frequently and there should be systematic updating.

- IT facilities for viewing and discussion of CVs and application forms with advisors.
- Storage for confidential files.
- Seminar room with audio-visual facilities for workshops. Overhead projectors are a minimum and PowerPoint projection is often required by medical speakers nowadays.

Optional but helpful

- IT facilities for clients to use independently to compose and improve CVs.
- Facilities for role play and feedback on interview skills, if possible with video recording and viewing facilities.
- Space for associated work towards career progress, such as mentoring, a PLAB study club.
- Book loan facility.
- Crèche.

Staffing

Careers advisors should be volunteer or paid medical practitioners, actively practising in the NHS. A project co-ordinator is required to oversee the scheme's development, implementation and ongoing executive management. Adequate administrative staffing is vital as medical practitioners have complex working timetables and are an expensive and scarce resource; their productivity should be maximised by spending most of it doing actual advice work and work generated from advice work that only they can do. Administration will include reception work as well as secretarial work and office management.

Both the medical careers advisors and the generic careers support personnel they work with will require some training. Medical advisors should be familiar with common or important aspects of their clients' needs that they may encounter and learn where to refer them appropriately for these. These may include psychological support, welfare assistance and immigration advice. It is important that medical advisors recognise their strengths, their roles and their limitations, otherwise it is easy to be caught up in the several other problems that the refugee doctor may also be facing.

The generic careers support personnel need to be aware that the medical career pathways are uniquely complex and competitive and have their own idiosyncrasies and customs. Incorrect advice can have serious consequences as it may be the sole source of information to someone who is desperate.

Accessing for users

Initial and ongoing publicity is important and this should be reviewed periodically to ensure all potential users who could benefit do hear of the service. It can be useful to ask new clients how they came to hear of the service, whether they actually needed to hear of it earlier on and how they may have been better reached. The information can be used to improve the publicity process as needed.

Funding and support

There are several agencies who might be approached for resources because the integration of refugee doctors into the NHS workforce could be part of their agenda. The resources might be in the form of money or practical support such as accommodation. These statutory or voluntary sector agencies can be considered under the following categories.

- Those with a career development/employment agenda, e.g. Jobcentre Plus.
- Those with an agenda to assist refugees with resettlement and integration, e.g. Home Office grants. Invitations for bids appear periodically on: www.ind. homeoffice.gov.uk/sitemap.asp
- Those with an agenda to develop services that reflect and thus better respond to the needs of refugees and migrants, e.g. the equalities department of the local strategic health authority.
- Those with an agenda for addressing recruitment needs in the NHS, e.g. workforce development confederations, soon to be absorbed into the strategic health authorities, and PCTs, particularly in areas of shortage such as is the case with GPs in inner cities.
- Those with an agenda for regeneration of areas, often urban regeneration, e.g. Single Regeneration Budgets (SRBs) operating in many cities in the UK.

Special considerations

Gender issues (with acknowledgement to Frances Lefford)

Refugee women doctors share the particular difficulties which face many women doctors. These may, however, be more severe and insurmountable because of the lack of a network of support and less understanding and access to information and forms of help in overcoming them.

Childcare poses a major problem, both financially and practically, and schemes need to include arrangements for this in their funding budgets. Options for overcoming this barrier include:

- providing a crèche on site during courses
- providing funding for childminding
- providing outreach services to community centres where voluntary child-care may be available
- prioritising women refugee doctors in training for local authority nursery places
- developing teaching tools that can be followed at home with telephone contact.

Domestic commitments can conflict with training courses and there is a need for flexibility in the timings of courses on offer. Those with school-age children may find mornings and early afternoons most appropriate, while others may find it easier to attend during evenings and weekends.

Women are more likely to be geographically restricted by family ties and may find it difficult to travel long distances to access training courses, clinical attachments or jobs.

Women may have lengthy gaps in their professional career path. Career breaks, which many UK women doctors take in order to raise a family, may be prolonged in the case of refugee women doctors through dislocation and the process of resettlement. Women in this position need to be given guidance on how to address this in the preparation of their CV and in job interviews.

Specialties

It is critical when advising refugee doctors to appreciate the very different pathways and opportunities existing in the different specialties at a given time and the likely future developments thereof. Any one consultant or GP will only have a ready familiarity with their own specialty. Junior doctors still at the stage of making their career path will be more familiar with the structures and possibilities more broadly, but are less likely to be employed in the career advisor role because of the nature of their clinical jobs at this stage. The ideal would be to have a group of career advisors available from a variety of specialties working together. The advisors are often unfortunately not available to do this. It is therefore important for medical careers advisors to keep abreast of the general training patterns and possibilities in the various specialties via the Royal Colleges and the deaneries.

The more competitive specialties find it very difficult to effectively differentiate between the hundreds of excellent candidates who may apply for a single senior house officer (SHO) post in their field. The consequence of this is that there seems to be less flexibility in the variety of candidates who will be accepted; the shortlist will be picked from those who fit the ideal candidate profile. This usually means a CV that demonstrates an early interest in the specialty, rapid progression through suitable posts for relevant experience, speedy acquisition of relevant postgraduate qualifications and a recent career history that guarantees they will walk in on their first day and be able to take on their duties and fit in with no hiccups. Increasing centralisation of the appointment systems has meant decreasing flexibility in this process to consider the non-standard candidate, who may have experience abroad that is more difficult to measure against that of locally grown applicants or who may have spent time away from their career for unconventional reasons such as war or resettlement. On the positive side, it has also brought transparency and the wider more effective application of equal opportunities policy so that candidates who may have previously been discriminated against on grounds of age should at least have a chance to get to the shortlist (if the date of graduation is not used against them).

The result of these conditions in the recruitment pathway of these competitive specialties is that experienced specialists, perhaps former consultants, in specialties such as surgery or dermatology find it impossible to work again in their field. They will often find it harder to get a job than a graduate from abroad who has never worked a day. Even when applying for SHO posts, they may be advised that they are overqualified and need to apply at a higher grade. Consultants considering their application often seem to empathise and feel that they themselves could not cope with working at that level again. However, they may not understand the very different viewpoint of a doctor who may have been living on benefits or doing unskilled work to whom simply to work with patients again would be a wonderful step forward. When applying for a higher grade they are advised that their lack of UK experience makes them unprepared to work and supervise juniors at that level. If they are able to adapt and are interested, they may be advised that a change of specialty may be the best way forward. Information about and, if possible, exposure by way of a clinical attachment to an unfamiliar specialty within an unfamiliar health service may assist in this decision. Some are not interested in working in another field and wish to pursue a highly competitive career against the odds. It should be remembered that people still do sometimes progress unexpectedly well, because they are outstanding or lucky, and they should be supported and given the chance if they want to try. The worst that can happen is that they fail in their chosen specialty and then choose another when they are ready. A judicious first step is to start in a specialty that can open the door to many other specialties, such as accident and emergency medicine.

The thorny problem of the doctor who may never again work as a doctor does arise sometimes. It can occur with the specialist of many years' standing, with the doctor who may have not practised for 10 years or the doctor who cannot pass the IELTS or PLAB exams. The difficulties in approaching this problem can be seen to arise from both the refugee doctor and the medical advisor. Medicine is always more than just a job. For most doctors it is truly a vocation: it gives unparalleled job satisfaction in the opportunity to serve and the challenge to several aspects of intelligence under pressure; it affords status and pays well. Wherever doctors come from, their qualifications have usually required competition and years of study to achieve. Initially for both the doctor advised and the medical advisor, a change from medicine can be seen as a terrible failure and loss. However, this also needs to be viewed as the opportunity to avoid a worse situation of not working or working far below potential capacity.

The decision to turn their back on medicine must be taken by the refugee doctors as they are the ones who may regret this and in any case doctors do sometimes exceed expectations and should be given some opportunity to try to do this if wished. Again the decision can be reversed later when the refugee doctor is ready. The choice of a new career outside medicine should rest on the needs, aspirations and abilities of the refugee doctor as well as the constraints of opportunities available. These factors must be honestly considered and assessed. Individual doctors may attach differing degrees of importance to contact with the public, public service ethos, social status, intellectual challenge and size of income. This will decide whether they are going to be happiest as physician's assistants, secondary school teachers, health service managers, medical researchers, drug industry representatives or by getting onto the graduate trainee programme of a bank.

How to set up and run a mentoring service (with acknowledgement to Kona Katembwe)

What is mentoring?

The Standing Committee on Postgraduate Medical and Dental Education defines mentoring in the following way:[3]

> 'An experienced highly regarded empathic person (the mentor) guides another individual (the mentee) in the development and re-examination of his or her own ideas, learning, personal and professional developments. This is achieved by listening and talking in confidence.'

The mentor assists the mentee to acquire new skills and insights and develop his or her full potential. People learn and develop most effectively by setting their own agenda, finding their own solutions at their own pace and making their own mistakes.[4] Mentoring schemes are increasingly being developed both within workplace settings and also in order to help people who are unemployed to enter the workforce. They are particularly relevant for refugee doctors who are seeking employment within a health service which is unfamiliar and who benefit greatly from 'signposting' and from support and guidance from someone who is highly familiar with the system.

Each mentoring relationship is unique and should reflect the needs and wishes of the two people within it. The relationship may change over time and may need to be re-evaluated. Not all of the mentee's needs may be met by an individual mentor.

In describing the characteristics of mentoring programmes, we do not intend to be prescriptive but rather to offer some suggestions for those who are thinking about developing a mentoring relationship.

Functions of mentoring

A mentoring relationship aims to promote self-development, build confidence and enhance creativity. It can provide teaching, support, advice, guidance, information on relevant resources and a role model. It can facilitate links to professional and networking relationships, which may otherwise not be accessible for the mentee.

Although the mentoring process is often looked upon as a one-way process with the mentee being the main beneficiary, current mentoring programmes tend to view mentoring as more of a two-way process in which both mentor and mentee benefit in terms of their self-development and professional enrichment. Thus it may be seen as more of a mutual relationship, with both mentor and mentee contributing and benefiting.

The mentor can develop skills in coaching and counselling,[4] a greater appreciation and understanding of issues through reflection and seeing them from another point of view, and considerable personal satisfaction. It may enhance a mentor's own career development and be relevant to appraisal.

Role of the mentor

A mentor can provide assistance in many ways including:[2,5]

- guiding the mentee in exploring career path options, discussing the various possibilities and signposting to additional sources of help and advice. A refugee doctor will need to know in which specialties he or she is likely to progress. Being usually somewhat older than UK-trained doctors applying for the same jobs, it is important not to have unreal expectations about progressing in a highly competitive specialty
- establishing trust in order to provide a confidential non-judgemental setting in which it is possible to discuss sensitive issues

- stimulating and extending the mentee's strengths, aspirations and potential
- motivating and supporting the mentee to develop ideas and take risks
- transferring skills and providing coaching for the mentee to develop them
- offering advice which is specially tailored to the mentee's particular situation
- assisting in setting realistic goals and targets
- introducing alternative views and options if it is apparent that the mentee's original goals are not possible. This needs to be handled sensitively and realistically. It may be particularly relevant in the case of older doctors, doctors who have been out of work for a very long period and those who are trained in a highly competitive specialty
- offering insight on a mentee's decisions and actions to assist understanding as to whether they are helpful
- assisting in developing job search and interview skills, including writing CVs
- giving specialist language support – increasing familiarity with medical terminology
- developing presentation skills
- keeping records for the purposes of monitoring and evaluation.

Box 12.1: Qualities needed to be a mentor (based on [4,5])

- Experience
- Respect for others' views
- Non-judgemental
- Belief that the mentee has the potential to succeed
- Willingness to have a supportive role without taking responsibility for decision making away from the mentee
- Preparedness to work with aspects of both professional and personal life
- Good communication skills: listening, giving and receiving feedback, questioning skills
- Approachability
- Ability to challenge constructively
- Flexibility
- Ability to encourage and inspire
- Networking skills
- Honesty
- Awareness of own competencies and limits with the willingness to seek help if necessary
- Willingness to allow the mentee to make own decisions
- Ability to positively support a mentee through the consequences of a decision

Background qualifications and recruitment of mentors

When recruiting mentors use should be made of local and national networks in order to advertise widely. Target your advertising to reach the right people.[6] Recruiting mentors may take several months. The mentor's role and terms and conditions need to be made clear, with a job description and person specification provided (for a model job description, see [2]), and whether the work is to be voluntary or paid should be made explicit. All applicants should provide references and interviews should be held to assess suitability.[6]

In our experience the input of a generalist careers advisor is important in assisting refugee doctors who are looking for help with their career development. However, the specialist knowledge that practising doctors can bring is something that refugee doctors find especially valuable.

Role of the mentee[4]

The mentee needs to commit to taking responsibility for developing objectives and goals, identify areas for self-learning and training needs and to complete actions identified with the mentor within an agreed timescale. The mentee can identify his or her strengths and weaknesses and experiment with new approaches and techniques.

Funding

Funding will be needed for the administrator's post. Mentees' expenses will need reimbursement and if mentors are working as volunteers, their expenses may also need to be reimbursed. Include childcare costs for mentees, who will also need funding to support their learning needs – books, courses, exam fees, etc.

Possible funding sources for mentoring schemes include the Department of Health or your local workforce development confederation.

Staff required

A mentoring scheme will need an administrator to organise recruitment of mentors and mentees, induction and ongoing training for mentors, co-ordination and administration of the scheme and support for both mentees and mentors. The administrator needs to be available if mentees or mentors have ongoing issues or problems which need to be addressed. The post may be full or part time depending on the size of the scheme. It may be advisable to have a steering group, with representation from refugee doctors. The administrator should be responsible for ensuring that the progress of the scheme undergoes regular review.

Training and support

Induction is important for both mentors and mentees, in order to explain the role and functioning of the mentoring scheme. This should form part of the recruitment and assessment process as attitudes or information may become apparent that influence whether the person is suitable to be a mentor.[6] As part of the training, mentors need to be made aware of the background context and situation of refugees and the challenges and barriers which they will be facing when trying to re-enter the job market. Training should also address the roles of the mentor and mentee and setting and maintaining boundaries.[6]

Although mentors will be paired as far as possible with mentees who match their own experience, it is also important for mentors to be familiar with the wide variety of medical careers and opportunities, including options for those who are unable to return to working as a doctor. Skills training may also be offered, such as listening and communication skills.[6]

A mentor needs to decide the amount of time he or she is willing to make available to a mentee for meeting face to face and whether further time will be made available in between for telephone and/or email contact.

Issues of confidentiality need to be made clear; as doctors, mentors will be familiar with the concept of confidentiality as it relates to patients. The same rules of confidentiality should be respected within the mentoring programme, i.e. information concerning a mentee should not be passed on to anyone without the consent of the mentee. Information about a mentee should only be shared with other people working within the programme on a 'need to know' basis, i.e. consider carefully who needs to know what and why. Records should be kept in a secure place and should only be accessed by authorised people. Both mentee and mentor should have access to written records which relate to them.

Matching

Each mentor would usually be matched with 1–2 mentees, depending on the time which they have available, and will be seeing them individually. It is preferable to match those who have the most in common professionally, i.e. match a surgeon with a surgeon, a primary care doctor with a GP (note, however, that the structure of primary care in the majority of countries from which refugees originate is very different from primary care in the UK).

It is also important to be aware of gender and cultural issues. There are particular challenges which may affect women and refugee women doctors may feel more comfortable with a female mentor. In some cultures an older person may find it hard to accept advice from a person who is much younger than them.

The initial meeting

Ideally, the first meeting of the mentor and mentee should take place with the person responsible for administration of the scheme also present. Expectations, ground rules and administrative arrangements can be made clear and any questions addressed, making clear how the administrator can be contacted in the future. A contract may be agreed although it may be more appropriate to discuss this at a subsequent meeting, once a relationship has been established.

The main purpose of the first meeting is to build trust between the mentee and mentor. Time is needed to get to know each other, feel comfortable and to form a trusting relationship. The mentee needs to think about what he or she wishes to gain from the relationship and the ways of achieving it.

Subsequent meetings

Meetings need to be at a time and place which are mutually convenient and the venue needs to offer privacy. It can be helpful to have a telephone, but this is not essential as calls can be made at another time. Sessions usually last 1–1.5 hours.

At the beginning there may be a need to meet more frequently (perhaps once a fortnight) but as the relationship develops, the time span between sessions can be increased to monthly and the use of other resources should be encouraged.[4] It needs to be agreed whether the mentee can contact the mentor between meetings by phone or email.

Goal or direction setting

The mentee should be encouraged to discuss and set goals, which may evolve as the relationship develops. Action points agreed at the end of each session can be helpful, so that it is clearly understood what the mentee and mentor have each agreed to do before the next session. The majority of these points should be the responsibility of the mentee, but the mentor may agree to make some telephone calls, find out some information, etc.

Mentoring aims to enable the mentee to develop through challenging their thinking and assisting them to identify the strengths and weaknesses of their ideas and their development needs.

Particular areas which may need addressing with refugee doctors include the following.[2]

- The NHS differs greatly from health systems in countries from which refugee doctors originate and, in addition to reading about its structure and function, it can be very helpful to have an explanation from a mentor who is actually working within it.
- The doctor–patient relationship is also very different in the UK and refugee doctors will benefit from acculturisation. Many patients expect more explanation concerning their medical care and mentees may have very different interpretations of issues such as confidentiality, particularly regarding confidentiality within families. Communication skills, including the breaking of bad news, can be addressed.
- Clinical attachments (*see* Chapter 9).
- Preparation for job applications, including writing CVs and interview techniques and practice.

Ongoing support

It can be very helpful for mentees to meet regularly with other mentees and for mentors to meet on a similar basis with other mentors. The purpose of these meetings is for mutual support, identifying challenges and ways of overcoming them and learning from different approaches. Both mentors and mentees can benefit by keeping a diary in order to reflect on their experiences and understanding better what works well.

Review

Regular reviews should be arranged to check that both mentor and mentee are finding the relationship useful and in order to learn from the experience. These can be formal or informal, but care should be taken to ensure that the mentee feels confident to express his or her views. Original goals should be reviewed in order to assess if these need updating.

Ending the mentoring relationship

Some mentees may only need a short relationship focusing on a particular goal, e.g. if they are successful in finding work quickly. Others may need a much longer mentoring relationship although, as has been stated before, it is likely that meetings will become less frequent. After obtaining a job, the mentee may wish to continue the relationship until he or she feels confident in the new role. If the mentee will be geographically distant, it may be possible to continue phone or email contact.

Emotional well-being and mental health

Refugee doctors may have experienced persecution in their country of origin, including violence, detention and torture. Many people experience symptoms commonly associated with post-traumatic experiences, including nightmares, intrusive thoughts, hypervigilance and feelings of anxiety.[7] Symptoms of anxiety, depression, guilt and shame and poor sleep patterns are very common. People may have problems with memory, concentration and disorientation, which hinder learning, including that of language. As well as being related to past experiences, these may also be related to people's current situation. Social isolation and poverty have a compounding effect, as do hostility and racism. Asylum seekers may be affected by uncertainty about their future and the fear of being sent home.[8]

For many, such experiences may be considered the natural expression of grief and distress concerning highly abnormal experiences and care should be taken not to pathologise. Common expressions of psychological and emotional distress do not necessarily mean the same in different cultural and social settings. For many people, restoration of their normal life as far as possible can be the most effective promoter of mental health and can do much to relieve feelings of sadness and anxiety.[9] In this respect, assisting refugee doctors to work again may greatly enhance their self-esteem and psychological well-being. Refugees have often survived against huge odds and their resilience may be a strength to be tapped into. Community and religious support may be important.

Some may welcome the opportunity to talk further and may benefit from referral to a counsellor. Many refugees wish to tell their story and find the process of testimony itself to be therapeutic, but it should not be assumed that people must do this in order to recover, and some find talking about their experiences extremely distressing and unhelpful.

In our experience, although a mentor could be expected to be supportive and empathic towards a mentee who is experiencing psychological difficulties, it is preferable not to mix the roles of mentor and counsellor. If a mentee is going through a particularly emotional time, they may wish to take a break from job seeking.

Symptoms that may need the involvement of specialist mental health services include:[9]

- consistent failure to function properly with daily tasks
- frequently expressed suicidal ideas or plans
- social withdrawal and self-neglect
- behaviour or talk that is abnormal or strange within the person's own culture
- aggression.

Table 12.1: Challenges and some possible solutions (based on [4])

Challenges/pitfalls	Possible solutions
Roles and responsibilities are unclear	Spend some time clarifying roles
Unsure what is meant to be achieved	Mentor and mentee should establish clear achievable aims, with an agenda for each session and action points
The mentee is passive and expects the mentor to come up with most of the suggestions	This may be due to the mentor being too directive; the mentor should aim to do more listening than talking
Mentor and mentee do not get on well together	Can you find ways to improve communication and find areas of common interest? If the relationship is still not working it may be necessary to find another mentor
Not finding the time to meet/cancelling sessions	May need help with time management
Mentee seems dependent on the mentor	At the start the mentor may need to give a lot of guidance and support but the aim should be to reduce this over time. The mentee's questions can be reflected to ask how he or she would deal with situations. A learning diary can be a useful way of reflecting on what has been learnt. A mentee should be supported to set the agenda and decide his or her own targets
Mentor feels uncomfortable challenging mentee	The mentor's training should include basic feedback skills. Balance positive with negative feedback
Mentor feels uncomfortable when mentee talks about personal matters	Mentor may need help with counselling skills or the mentee may need to find counselling support from elsewhere (note caution about combining roles of counsellor and mentor)

Monitoring and evaluation[5]

Evaluation is important in order to measure the effectiveness of the mentoring scheme and to make further improvements. It may be part of the funding agreement and will be useful when applying for future funding. Costs permitting, it may be useful to employ an external evaluator to provide an objective view. Interviews can be conducted with mentees, mentors and other relevant people, e.g. employers.

Quantitative information can include the number of meetings between mentors and mentees, costs, etc. Evaluating a mentoring relationship qualitatively could include:

- looking at the objectives and goals of the meetings and assessing whether they were useful and whether the meetings have been useful (process)
- asking the mentee the extent to which they could set the agenda and whether they felt they received honest feedback (communication)
- assessing whether the mentee is progressing and developing and is working towards the achievement of their goals (outcome)
- what aspects of the scheme have been helpful (and conversely which aspects have been less helpful)
- seeking suggestions for improvement from mentees, mentors and others.

References

1   Ward C and Eccles S (2001) *So You Want to be a Brain Surgeon.* Oxford University Press, Oxford.

2   Katembwe K and Prince B (2003) *A Guide to Mentoring Refugee Doctors.* RETAS, London.

3   Standing Committee on Postgraduate Medical and Dental Education (1998) *Supporting Doctors and Dentists at Work – an enquiry into mentoring.* SCOPME, London.

4   Hertfordshire TEC (1999) *Mentor's Handbook.* Herts TEC, St Albans.

5   Grainger C (2002) Mentoring – supporting doctors at work and play. *BMJ.* **324**: S203.

6   Wilson R (2003) *The A–Z of Volunteering and Asylum – a handbook for managers.* National Centre for Volunteering and Tandem Communications and Research, London.

7   Burnett A and Thompson K (2004) Enhancing the psychological well-being of asylum seekers and refugees. In: K Barrett and B George (eds) *Race, Culture, Psychology and Law.* Sage Publications, California.

8   Burnett A (2003) Care of refugees and asylum seekers. In: J Kai (ed) *Ethnicity, Health and Primary Care.* Oxford University Press, Oxford.

9   Burnett A and Fassil Y (2002) *Meeting the Health Needs of Refugees and Asylum Seekers in the UK: an information and resource pack for health workers.* London Directorate for Health and Social Care/Department of Health, London.

Resources

RETAS (Refugee Education and Advisory Service)
Education Action International
14 Dufferin Street
London EC1Y 8PD
Tel: 020 7426 5800 (general), 020 7426 5801 (advice)
Fax: 020 7251 1314
Email: retas@education-action.org
Website: www.education-action.org
RETAS runs a mentoring service for refugee doctors and is recruiting volunteer doctors as mentors. For further information contact Kona Katembwe on 020 7426 5800.

Katembwe K and Prince B (2003) *A Guide to Mentoring Refugee Doctors.* RETAS, London.
Includes background information on refugees' legal status and entitlements, understanding the asylum process, entitlement to education and training, financial support for higher education, educational trusts and charities, entitlements to employment.

Mentor's Handbook.
Herts TEC
45 Grosvenor Road
St Albans
Herts AL1 3AW
Tel: 01727 813600
Fax: 01727 813443
Email: info@herts.tec.co.uk
Website: www.herts.tec.co.uk
Includes information on the roles of mentors and mentees, benefits to both, challenges and pitfalls and further resources. It is not written specifically for mentoring refugee doctors but the information is transferable and relevant.

Grainger C (2002) Mentoring – supporting doctors at work and play. *BMJ.* **324**: S203.
Explains what a mentor is, how to choose one and what the mentoring relationship involves.

Wilson R (2003) *The A–Z of Volunteering and Asylum – a handbook for managers.* National Centre for Volunteering and Tandem Communications and Research, London.

Mentor Training Pack produced by Edinburgh Homeless Project
Website: www.homeless-ecsh.org

Refugee Council Training and Employment Section
Tel: 020 7346 6760
Email: training @refugeecouncil.org.uk

Mentors Forum
Website: www.mentorsforum.co.uk

National Mentoring Network
Website: www.nmn.org.uk

CHAPTER 13

Developing alternative roles for refugee doctors

Diana Cliff and John Eversley

'The Road that I follow
Leads me on my way
Got my eyes on tomorrow
And my feet on today.'
(JB Arthur, Steve McEwan and Nic Paton.
Sung by Miriam Makeba who spent
many years in exile from South Africa)

Refugee doctors have always worked in a wide range of jobs, usually low paid and low skilled. In the NHS, we are slowly waking up to the fact that refugee doctors have skills that we are desperately short of and that are underutilised. Many refugee doctors will go on to work as doctors in the UK but whilst they are preparing for their exams to requalify in the UK, they are working as cleaners, minicab drivers, in factories and petrol stations. A minority are working in hospitals as porters, phlebotomists, healthcare assistants and lab technicians. Some refugee doctors may never return to practising medicine. Many in the NHS are now asking the question: 'How can we use their skills in alternative ways?'. Refugee doctors themselves ask: 'What can I do to use and enhance my skills while I am not recognised? What alternative is there if I am not recognised?'.

This chapter will look at the work refugee doctors are doing and their views about it. It will also examine how the NHS is beginning to recognise and use the skills of refugee doctors to meet the huge demands of delivering an effective healthcare system for our diverse population of patients. It is early days; most of the doctors we have met (who are not yet practising as doctors) are not using their skills and express great dissatisfaction with their work. A small number have found meaningful work; this is often through opportunism and chance meetings with the right people rather than through a systematic recruitment programme. We will, however, present examples of structured programmes that are being developed and which enable healthcare employers to utilise the skills of refugee doctors.

When is a doctor not a doctor . . . ?

All the doctors we have worked with aspire to practise as doctors in the UK; the vast majority state that they are aiming and intending to do so. However, the majority of refugee doctors in the UK are unable to fulfil this aim.

The need to earn a wage to support themselves and their families is the motivation for most refugee doctors to work in non-clinical jobs. One doctor from Kosovo worked long hours for three years in manual work to send money back home to rebuild the family house for his mother and family. When this task was complete, he was able to concentrate on studying for his exams. Having a young family to support, he now works part time as a phlebotomist whilst training to requalify as a doctor in the UK.

Many doctors are frustrated because they cannot find even low-skilled work. They are often told they don't have the right background or are 'overqualified'. One doctor applied unsuccessfully for healthcare assistant jobs; when he asked why he was not successful, he was told that he didn't have any relevant experience. His years working as a doctor and his obviously compassionate manner did not count. He applied for a job as a mental health support worker but again was unsuccessful; he was told that he was 'used to higher level work'. 'What do I have to do?' he asked.

Another doctor was keen to find a job that would improve his skills, in particular his language skills. He had been studying English and claiming Job Seekers Allowance. After a year he was referred to New Deal and asked what job he could do. 'What about care assistant?' he suggested. 'You are not eligible, you need an NVQ to be a care assistant,' replied the job centre officer. 'You could work as a domestic assistant, that would be all right for you.' The doctor thought to himself, 'I can't say that I don't want to work,' so he replied, 'OK, I will start a domestic job'. He has now been working as a cleaner for several months and doing a general jobsearch course as part of the New Deal programme. The job centre was unable to find any hospital jobs on their database. The doctor sat for his English exam (IELTS) and got a lower grade than his previous attempt before he had been working.

The economic arguments are clear – such doctors will contribute more to society, including tax revenues, if they are allowed to retrain as doctors. Long acknowledged by government officials and politicians alike, a solution to this simple issue of doctors claiming benefits and being forced to take low-skilled, unrelated jobs rather than retrain as doctors has not yet been found.

A pilot scheme in north-east London is bringing together Jobcentre Plus and local NHS trusts, ensuring that healthcare vacancies are advertised in local job centres. Trusts will start focusing on competencies for jobs rather than qualifications. The aim is for trusts to recruit local people, including those from refugee communities, and to raise the awareness of job centre staff about jobs in health.

The doctors we have met want jobs 'to go forward', as one doctor puts it. Another said they want to improve their skills, particularly English skills.

Is there a doctor in the house?

Work in the NHS has the advantage of allowing doctors to find out how the NHS works, but few are fortunate enough to find work in health.

Some doctors from the old Soviet Union, including those from African countries such as Somalia and Ethiopia who had agreements with USSR countries, qualified as nurses before continuing their training as doctors. These doctors often find they can requalify and find work as a nurse more easily. One such doctor worked for several years as a nurse in accident and emergency. He did not tell his colleagues that he had actually trained as a doctor, until his story was featured in the local newspaper and pinned on a staff noticeboard.

Many of the phlebotomists in our hospitals are refugee doctors studying for their exams. It is a 'very dirty job' said one doctor who was reluctant to do it but needed the money. Others say it allows them to be part of the hospital, to visit all areas of the hospital and, according to one doctor, '(it's) OK as job for doctor as it's our work, it's with patients, I improve my English listening and speaking'.

Some refugee and overseas qualified doctors are working in GP surgeries. One doctor, a GP from Nigeria, came to this country in the 1970s and worked in Scotland in psychiatry for several years. He returned to Nigeria to look after his dying mother, remaining there just long enough to lose his full GMC registration. On his return, he struggled with the IELTS English exam even though he was a fluent English speaker – he speaks softly, slowly and with a Nigerian accent. Eventually gaining straight 7s in IELTS and qualifying for the now extinct 'senior doctor' route, he was eligible to get a job in psychiatry. Fate seemed against him. On being offered one job, the Home Office lost his passport. One agency offered him a job to start the next day in another part of the country; unable to move so fast, he lost the job as someone else was able to move quicker. He had been working for the last few years as a support worker with people with learning difficulties, when a project for refugee and overseas-qualified health professionals put him in touch with the local PCT which were aiming to train overseas-qualified health professionals as cardiovascular health technicians to meet coronary heart disease targets. The Nigerian doctor is now in his first year of the training; he is working full time in a GP surgery, a large training practice, from 8.30 to 6.30, taking the minimum holiday 'because it is a statutory requirement'. His work in the surgery is mainly carrying out new patient health checks and submitting paperwork on behalf of the GPs – forms needed to help patients claim insurance, sick pay, incapacity benefit, etc. He also spends a fair amount of his time doing reception work and endless piles of filing. Occasionally one of the GPs emerges and asks him to do some photocopying. Once a month he attends a local university to prepare for an NVQ in Care, funded by the local PCT. Others on the course include an Egyptian dentist, a Sri Lankan pharmacist and nurses from Somalia and the Ukraine. One cannot help but wonder how much more these health professionals could be contributing to primary care with a little training. Yet this potentially successful, innovative programme has had difficulty in accessing funding to provide additional supervision and training.

Alternative medicine

The contribution of refugee doctors to the health of their often isolated, excluded communities goes unmeasured. One doctor volunteers as a health adviser for his local Congolese church. A health project was set up out of concern about access to health services by their community. Stories of difficulties being able to register with GPs and getting referrals to consultants are commonplace, together with a lack of understanding within communities about the treatments advised by GPs. These difficulties often stem from language problems as well as cultural differences around health and treatment. The health project wanted to employ one of the doctors from their community to be a link between themselves and the health professionals and thereby address these issues. They approached the local PCT and the (then) health authority for support and funding, but were turned down. The refugee doctor in question speaks good English but has so far not met the high English requirements for GMC registration. He wants to be more than an advocate in assisting his community whilst accepting that he cannot prescribe and work as a doctor without registration. Having worked as a gynaecologist for 10 years, he recently held a meeting of Congolese women, to explain how intervention in the delivery of babies is managed in this country and to address some of the concerns of the women, such as the large percentage of babies being delivered through Caesarian section. The perception of the women was that it is due to staff shortages. Those who attended the meeting expressed a need for a Congolese link worker who understood the medical system in the UK. This illustrates that in the new NHS, where patient choice is key, patient needs are still left unmet but could be met with the help of refugee healthcare professionals.

Until there are more doctors and link workers from refugee communities in the NHS, the isolation of refugee communities and the negative consequences for their health will continue and we will hear examples of refugees failing to give informed consent for serious operations. One Somali doctor told of visiting another Somali woman in hospital. She had heard about her situation through a friend. The woman had undergone a hysterectomy without having understood what was happening until after the operation. In her culture, removal of the womb was unheard of and left her questioning her status as a woman.

One way of legitimising this voluntary work within the community is for doctors to gain alternative, non-clinical qualifications and find paid employment, e.g. in health promotion, public health or advocacy, as many have done. One Somali gynaecologist with a UK Masters in Health Promotion trains health workers on female genital mutilation. Another Somali gynaecologist runs a clinic for the local refugee community at a community health project. Often this work is sessional and only becomes possible after many years of working as a volunteer, with volunteers serving an unofficial 'apprenticeship'. Another refugee doctor works full time in health promotion for a PCT and is struggling to find time to study for the PLAB exam.

Of the refugee doctors who work as advocates, the authors know none who have returned to practising medicine. Unlike many of the other jobs that refugee doctors do, those who become advocates often report that it is a satisfying job. Many are contented in their new role but all still aspire to return to practising medicine.

Working differently

Many managers and clinicians in the NHS are looking at new ways of using the skills of refugee doctors, often by creating new roles. Often the answers to the shortage of GPs or hospital doctors is to train nurses to take on a wider range of responsibilities. But there is also a shortage of nurses. In the NHS, we therefore need to look at new pools of labour – from science graduates to ex-army medical personnel and, of course, refugee doctors.

English workforce development confederations recently reported that the 'NHS will have to compete very hard if it is to retain an overall workforce of about 1.2 million people – let alone grow it by about 300 000'.[1] They report that 'Any workforce expansion policy that is driven by attracting an ever growing percentage of an ever shrinking population of school, college and university leavers is doomed to failure'. This work highlights the shortage of applicants to higher-level vacancies in the NHS but says, 'It is interesting to ask (NHS managers) how many applications they receive for jobs such as healthcare assistants or trainee ambulance personnel' – the numbers often exceed 100 for just one vacancy. The report states that 'A systematic approach to large-scale workforce modernisation involving increased reliance on staff who are not registered professionals ... will be (a) significant part of the answer. This means many more assistant practitioners'. In parts of the country (Birmingham, Manchester, Bristol, Newcastle, Glasgow, etc.) where there are significant numbers of refugee health professionals unable to return directly to their professions, they have a ready supply of ideal applicants for these jobs.

For those refugee doctors who are aware they might not return to medicine, the new roles of physician's assistants are an exciting development with great potential. One doctor who is working as an intensive care nurse said he would like to have a role more akin to his original work, such as a physician's assistant.

In the US, physician's assistants have a key role in healthcare delivery, with a three-year dedicated degree course as the entry point. Tipton PCT in the Midlands has recruited three physician's assistants from the US to work in GP surgeries and is exploring how they could employ home-grown recruits. The University of Hertfordshire is introducing a one-year postgraduate degree course firstly to train nurses who want to be physician's assistants and a two-year course for others such as science graduates. There could be a similar route for refugee health professionals, ideally part time so they could be employed and study at the same time.

In Slough, one practice is using two overseas-qualified doctors to work with their growing number of asylum seeker patients. The two doctors carry out patient histories and examinations and check the diagnosis with the GP who then writes the prescription if appropriate.

Dr Nayeem Azim's College of North Central London trained a number of refugee doctors as unpaid GP support workers. Some doctors continue as practice employees carrying out phlebotomy, taking and reading ECGs, completing new patient health checks, taking and monitoring blood pressure and cholesterol levels, as well as dealing with routine paperwork.

The role of the physician's assistant, which offers great potential for the NHS, is now being explored. In the acute sector, physician's assistant is being used by some hospitals to refer to a job which seems to combine healthcare assistant duties with administrative duties. We need to incorporate a Skills Escalator approach, ensuring that refugee doctors have the opportunity to progress through a range of jobs with increasing levels of responsibility.

Many refugee doctors working in health have come to their jobs through volunteering and being in the right place at the right time. One well-connected doctor who had worked in medicine across the world, including work with the Red Cross, was invited to lecture on a global health programme at his local university. Another chance meeting, with the Chief Executive of his local WDC, led him to a job co-ordinating work with refugee health professionals in his area. But we should not trust to luck in converting this potential workforce into an appropriately utilised supply.

The road to follow

The fact is that all the doctors we met want to return to medicine and it is as doctors that the NHS needs them. In looking at alternative work for refugee doctors, we need to see it as both a route to becoming a doctor and as a valued alternative career incorporating a Skills Escalator approach.

There are a number of ways in which this might be achieved.

1 *Review entry requirements.* With all the jobs and training possibilities described above, recruitment and admissions staff should consider carefully job specifications and entry requirements. 'Lack of UK experience' or 'overqualification' is generally unjustifiable discrimination under UK race relations law. NHS Professionals, Job Centres Plus and workforce development confederations have a key role in making sure that employers and colleges do not discriminate.
2 *Giving support.* Although there are a variety of refugee health professional support agencies, there are still gaps. When a refugee doctor experiences discrimination, ignorance, incompetence or maladministration, the agencies that know most about healthcare, employment or higher education rules are not necessarily the same as those who know most about refugees. There is a need for collaboration between, for instance, the Medical Defence Union and refugee advice agencies.
3 *Combine study and public services.* Unrecognised doctors need financial support while studying for their PLAB and they have linguistic, cultural and clinical knowledge that make them valuable in a variety of roles, such as GP support assistants, phlebotomists and care assistants. More and better opportunities of this kind could be developed. A template for job descriptions, person specifications and working arrangements is needed. Workforce development confederations could provide training courses for such posts.
4 *Create pathways to alternative careers.* The jobs above do not necessarily offer much opportunity for progression. Physician's assistants posts, for instance, could address the shortage of nurses as well as doctors. The nursing background that many refugee doctors have gives them additional skills to offer. Greater clarification and development of the physician's assistant role are needed. Application of the concept of skills escalators is essential.
5 *Teaching and research.* Work in universities in teaching and research offers an opportunity to keep in touch with medical developments as well as to contribute in areas of expertise such as global health. Orientation and skills development in learning and teaching methods will be necessary for some doctors.
6 *Public health* in the UK is changing. Increased emphasis on community-led needs assessment and patient profiling creates opportunities for doctors to practise non-clinically. There is a range of postgraduate public health opportunities that may be useful.
7 *Community and voluntary work.* Unpaid work is often both an inevitable part of being a refugee doctor and an opportunity. They are called on:

- for diagnostic advice
- to recommend over-the-counter remedies and explain their use and contraindications
- to accompany members of their community to health appointments
- to explain to other healthcare professions community needs and perceptions.

All these roles can be legitimate and desirable but there are also legal and common-sense rules and standards that need to be followed. As well as rules on what only recognised health professionals can do, there are also rules about voluntary work for asylum seekers, for example. Refugee health projects should take responsibility for making sure these rules are followed and understood by healthcare providers too.

8   *Health promotion.* As well as specific opportunities in working with refugee communities, health promotion offers more general career opportunities. There are postgraduate training opportunities to assist entry to health promotion jobs, now often located in primary care trusts but also in voluntary organisations.

9   *Work with children.* A number of refugee doctors are already trained as paediatricians and many others will have worked with children. Learning assistants in schools, Surestart programmes and multiagency child protection programmes all offer opportunities. Criminal Records Bureau checks will be required. They tend to take longer for people who have come to the UK.

References

1   Sargent J (2003) *A Proposal to Develop a National Framework for Assistant Practitioners and Advanced Practitioners.* Standing Conference of English WDC Chief Executives, London.

Appendix: support for other refugee health professionals

Diana Cliff

Introduction

Much work is taking place across the country with refugee nurses. Internationally qualified nurses have always been a key part of the workforce of the NHS and there are large numbers of refugee nurses who would like to work as nurses in the NHS. The British Dental Association has also been proactive in initiating support for refugee dentists and there is a significant amount of work developing around the UK.

At the time of writing (September 2003), there is little proactive work with refugee pharmacists, allied health professionals and medical scientists and hence the routes for these professionals appear to be quite blocked although some individuals are successful if their qualifications are similar to UK qualifications, they show persistence and have access to financial resources.

One of the difficulties in setting up support for refugee health professionals other than doctors and nurses is that the numbers are small and they are dispersed across the country as well as across London. Partnerships set up to support refugee doctors and nurses are slowly beginning to look at how best to support other refugee health professionals get through the requalification process and into the NHS.

Nurses and midwives

Requalification routes for refugee nurses and midwives

To register with the Nursing and Midwifery Council (NMC), refugee nurses and midwives need to complete an application process (involving references from their college of nursing/midwifery, employers and registration bodies as well as a transcript of training). Once they have received a decision from the NMC about the appropriateness of their prior training and experience, most refugee nurses/midwives need:

- IELTS General Level 6.5, with a minimum score of 5.5 in each section, if they have trained in a language other than English
- a period of supervised practice for nurses, usually 3–6 months, or a period of adaptation for midwives, usually 6–12 months.

Contact details

Nursing and Midwifery Council (NMC)
23 Portland Place
London W1B 1PZ
Website: www.nmc-uk.org

Support for refugee nurses

Royal College of Nurses (RCN)

The RCN has a database of refugee nurses. Nurses on the database receive regular newsletters giving details of news, events and programmes throughout the country for refugee nurses.
  The RCN provides:

- career development workshops for refugee nurses
- refugee nurses' discussion group including guest speakers and discussion of member issues
- one-to-one careers.

Contact details

Royal College of Nursing
20 Cavendish Square
London W1G 0RN
Website: www.rcn.org.uk/news/refugeenurses.php

Refugee Nurses Taskforce

The taskforce is made up of 24 members representing all major stakeholders, from the NHS and independent sector, workforce development confederations, professionals organisations and unions, government departments and Jobcentre Plus, training providers and the voluntary sector, the Refugee Council and Praxis.

Their aim is to identify practical solutions to the barriers facing refugee nurses in accessing: accurate information and advice; communications skills training; orientation, adaptation and supervised practice programmes; statutory registration for practice and jobs and career progression and pathways. They are due to report back to a wider group of stakeholders in mid 2004.

Example of good practice: Praxis Community Project

Praxis is a community-led organisation with expertise in working with refugee nurses. They offer advice and guidance for refugee nurses and midwives, as well as other refugee health professionals, and preparation for supervised practice courses for refugee and local overseas-qualified nurses. Courses include:

- communication and numeracy including colloquial language, nursing and medical terminology
- familiarity with the NHS and preparing nurses to enter the NHS working environment
- nursing care in the UK.

A similar course is being developed for midwives who live in north-east London.

Financial assistance to individual refugees, public relations, research and learning materials development are also available.

Contact details

Praxis
Pott Street, off Bethnal Green Road
London E2 0EF
Tel: 020 7729 7985
Website: www.praxis.org.uk

Other projects for nurses

There are several projects around the country supporting refugee nurses including those in the north-east of England, Glasgow, Midlands, Manchester, Bristol and Cardiff. Contact the RCN whose newsletter gives full details.

Dentists

Requalification route for dentists – to register with the General Dental Council (GDC)

To get full registration dentists must take the IELTS exam and must achieve a score of at least 7 in all four components before they can take the GDC's International Qualifying Exam (IQE).

The IQE has three parts.

- Part A comprises written and oral examinations in basic sciences and human diseases and an oral examination in clinical dentistry.
- Part B consists of an operative test on a dental manikin.
- Part C contains written examinations in all aspects of dentistry, an examination in clinical dentistry and an examination in medical emergencies.

For more information, see the GDC website.

Refugee dentists are also eligible for temporary registration without taking the IQE. Temporary registration allows them to do postgraduate studies and dental attachments. They should contact the NACPDE for more details – *see* below.

To become a general dental practitioner, dentists must pass the IQE to be eligible for full registration and then apply for a vocational training which involves one year working as a vocational training practitioner in a general dental surgery.

Contact details

General Dental Council
37 Wimpole Street
London W1M 8DQ
Tel: 020 7887 3800
Website: www.gdc-uk.org

British Dental Association (BDA)

The BDA and the Refugee Council have established a database of refugee and asylum seeker dentists. They send out to everyone on the database a newsletter every three months which gives details of courses, funding and other support mechanisms.

Free membership of the BDA is available to refugee dentists who have Indefinite Leave to Remain (refugee status) or Exceptional Leave to Remain and a letter from the GDC confirming their eligibility for temporary registration.

The BDA is piloting a mentoring scheme.

The BDA and the Refugee Council have also established a Refugee Dentist Steering Group which lobbies and liaises with other organisations on behalf of refugee dentists.

Contact details

BDA
64 Wimpole Street
London W1G 8YS
Tel: 020 7563 4140
Website: www.bda-dentistry.org.uk

National Advice Centre for Postgraduate Dental Education (NACPDE)

Provides information and advice on all aspects of postgraduate training mainly to refugee and overseas-qualified dentists.

Contact details

Faculty of Dental Surgery
Royal College of Surgeons of England
35–43 Lincoln's Inn Fields
London WC2A 3PE
Tel: 020 7869 6804
Website: www.rcseng.ac.uk/dental/fds/nacpde

Postgraduate deaneries

Deaneries around the country (for example, in London, the North West, Merseyside and Newcastle) are starting to set up support to facilitate the access of refugee dentists through the requalification process.

Example of good practice: Pan London Refugee Dentists Study Group

A group of organisations working with refugee health professionals across London got together to establish a study group for refugee dentists. This is now held weekly in Ladbroke Grove and is facilitated by a dental educationalist.

Contact details

Refugee and Migrant Communities Forum
2 Thorpe Close
London W10 5XL
Tel: 020 8964 4815

Pharmacists

Requalification route for refugee pharmacists

Refugee pharmacists must apply to the Royal Pharmaceutical Society (RPS). To be eligible, pharmacists must have completed a pharmacy course that is comparable to those in the UK and must be registered or eligible to register as a pharmacist overseas.

The RPS requires overseas-qualified pharmacists to have an IELTS academic level score of 7 in each of the sections.

After the Society's preliminary consideration of a pharmacist's documentation, they may be given the standard Adjudicating Committee requirements which are:

- to successfully complete the Overseas Pharmacists (OSP) Assessment Programme
- to complete 12 months pre-registration training
- to pass the Society's registration examination.

Alternatively, pharmacists may be required to attend a formal interview before the Committee and if accepted, complete the above process of OSP, pre-registration training and the Society's exam.

The OSP is currently held at Sunderland University with fees of £7300 which may be reduced to £1000 for those who qualify as home students. Those with refugee status or those with Exceptional Leave to Remain (ELR) who have been in the UK for three years may be considered as home students and eligible to apply for a student loan from their local authority.

The application and interview fee for the RPS is waived for refugees and those with ELR and is refunded to those who receive their settled status from the Home Office at a later date.

Overseas-qualified pharmacists must also have an IELTS score of 7.

For more information, get a copy of the RPS's information pack.

The various refugee health professionals projects around the country that are supporting refugee doctors and nurses, may also support refugee pharmacists, e.g. with financial support for exam fees, travel expenses, etc.

Many overseas-qualified pharmacists find work as pharmacy assistants whilst they are settling in the UK.

One of the main barriers for refugee pharmacists is that the only conversion course is held in Sunderland and the costs of the fees and expenses.

Contact details

Overseas Registration
Royal Pharmaceutical Society of Great Britain
1 Lambeth High Street
London SE1 7JN
Tel: 020 7572 2317
Website: www.rpsgb.org

Allied health professionals and medical scientists

Requalification route for refugee AHPs

Allied health professionals (AHPs) and medical scientists should apply for registration to the Health Professionals Council (HPC).

The Professional Boards assess the qualifications and experience of overseas-qualified AHPs and medical scientists in comparison to UK-trained professionals. They look at information provided by the applicant's referees, their training institutions and any education, training and experience provided in the application. There are several possible outcomes to the assessment process.

- Acceptance to the Register.
- Rejection due to insufficient basic levels of training and qualifications.
- Rejection but with opportunities to join the Register following further training, experience or adaptation. Note there may be a time limit on these.
- Request further verification or invitation to attend a Test of Competence based on the professions' Standards of Proficiency.

The HPC requires overseas-qualified AHPs and health scientists (who did not train in English) to have an IELTS academic level score of 7 (with a minimum score of 6.5 in each section) with speech and language therapists required to have an academic level of 8.0 (with a minimum score of 7.5 in each section).

The main barrier for refugee AHPs and medical scientists is that their overseas qualifications are often not accepted by the HPC as similar to a UK qualification and it is recommended that they undertake UK pre-registration training.

Support for AHPs and medical scientists

Many of the projects supporting refugee health professionals will support AHPs and medical scientists in the same way, by providing advice, advocacy, IELTS courses and funding. However, many organisations are less knowledgeable about the routes for AHPs and medical scientists. At the time of writing (September 2003) we know of no specific projects to support refugee AHPs although WDCs and voluntary sector advice agencies in London are in the process of establishing new initiatives.

Contact details

Health Professionals Council
Park House
184 Kennington Park Road
London SE11 4BU
Tel: 020 7582 0866
Website: www.hpc-uk.org

Index

Page numbers in italics refer to tables.

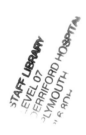